WALK AGAINST TIME

One Girl's Journey

in the

Breast Cancer 3-Day

a novel

by

Paul Wake Baker

This is a work of fiction. Names, characters, businesses, places, events, locales, and incidents are either the products of the author's imagination or used in a fictitious manner. Any resemblance to actual persons, living or dead, is purely coincidental.

WALK AGAINST TIME

Sod House Press, LLC

Model: Jacklyn Strahan.
Team photo uncredited.

Book design and maps by Paul Wake Baker, Copyright 2021.
Map ink by Ben Fry.

Sod House Press, LLC
Lincoln, Nebraska

Visit our web site at: www.sodhousepress.com
Visit the author's web site at: www.paulwakebaker.com

Printed in the United States of America

ISBN: 978-0-578-24723-6

Dedication

This book is for Ann Moss, Mary Elizabeth Rea, Patti Solis, Deidre Rhinehart, Sieglinde Schmid, and many others whose lives were taken by breast cancer. It is also in acknowledgement of the survival of Katie Ohnoutka, Ashleigh Rhinehart, Rae Lovell, and many others. And last of all, it is dedicated gratefully to all of the members of the real Team Aquatic Park, but especially to Kevan & Pat Curren, Jennifer Baus, Natalie and Mike, Christine, Ed & Nancy & Scooter, Kris, Lisa, Dean & MJ, Terry, Carol & Stephanie Smith, Marjorie, Megan Keene, Susan Schaeffer, Taya, Pat, Amy, Rolando, Cindra, Jeff, Janice, Alicia, Page, Liz, Lori, Faren, Matthew, Rene, Dara, Kelli, Yolanda, Giz, Freddie, Mara, and anyone else I may have accidentally left out. I truly appreciate your contribution. Also grateful thanks to Glen and all of the members of the San Jose Police who volunteered their time for the safety of the walkers.

Team Aquatic Park

Although *Walk Against Time* is a work of fiction, I extend my deepest thanks to the **real members of Team Aquatic Park** and all of those who trained with us. Your work and dedication in both 2000 and 2001 was inspirational. Thank you!

Those fond memories led me to write this novel and I hope that at least part of this fictitious story represents the reality of our experiences and I hope you will forgive me for making David Cook a much better leader than I. It's my fondest hope that this novel will inspire others in the fight to end breast cancer.

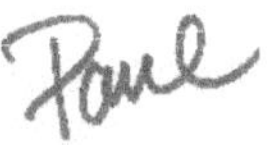

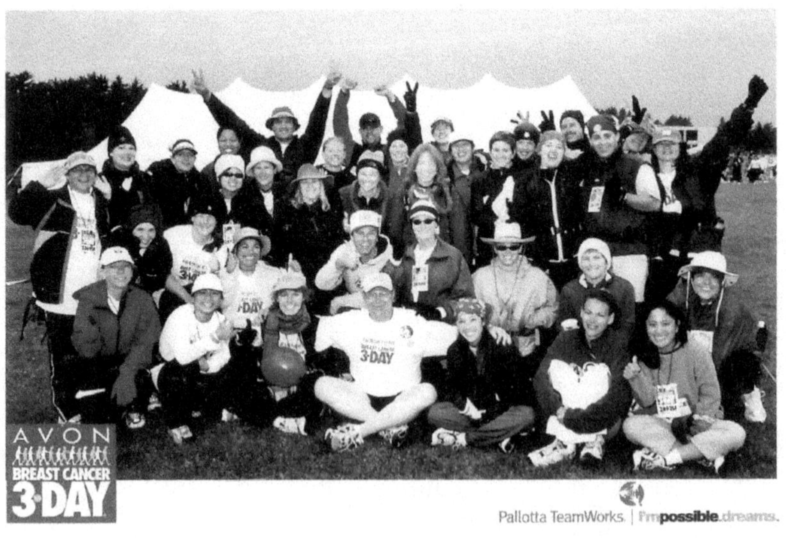

TRAINING WALK MAPS

Instructions on page opposite map

1

Training Journal of Emmy Wells

1/26	Friday	3 Miles, Embarcadero, Pier 39.
1/27	Saturday	5 Miles, Fulton St./Cliff House.

January 28, 2001, 4:28 am

Man, oh, man, what a way to start my first official day of training! I just woke up from another Amy nightmare. It was right before she died—my last visit to California Pacific. I was walking up the sidewalk and saw Grace sitting on the bench outside. She was crying and I knew then—I knew that Amy was going to die—and then everything went black. Just like before. I can't remember what happened.

But I *do* remember the panic—the worst I've ever felt in my life.

Scary as hell.

Anyway, I've got to shake it off. In a few hours I'm going to my first official Training Walk.

Since January 2nd—when Tina signed me up—I've walked a few

miles a day during lunch and more on weekends—up to 5 miles in one walk. That's why I decided to start this journal. It's mostly to keep track of miles, but it also gives me a chance to vent about how much I hate what I'm doing without inflicting it on others. So here goes:

1. Every day, my lower back, calves, thighs, feet—and even my butt—ache with pain. I haven't done shit yet and I'm hurting all the time.
2. As if physical pain isn't bad enough, I've spent over $300 on shoes, socks, shorts, sports bras, and tops. And two fanny packs: one XL (I call it the Blowfish) and the other tiny (the Minnow).
3. I had to sit through an hour of orientation listening to a guy from Pallotta TeamWorks—the co-sponsor of the event with Avon—evangelize about raising the minimum requirement of $1,900.

"We want you to *double* it!" he said. "Or *triple* it!"

Man! I don't want to ask people for money! Hell, I don't even want to be doing this.

If it wasn't for Tina—no, I can't blame Tina. This little exercise in physical and economic torture is the brainchild of Dr. Barbara ("Call me Barb!") Jenner.

Her idea of therapy is to fill my life with positive things to do. You would think classes in the morning and work in the afternoon would be way plenty, but no, she wanted me to start walking. That's all, just walk. Then she brought a newspaper ad for the Breast Cancer 3-Day to one of our sessions and held it up in front of me like a bullfighter.

"This is perfect for you!" she said. "Think about it. You can do something for your aunt."

That *really* pissed me off. It's too late to do *anything* for Amy and she knows it. Even so, I brought the ad to work, Tina saw it, got psyched, and before I knew it I'd signed up to walk 60 miles from San Jose to San Francisco—in July no less. The Avon Frickin' Breast Cancer 3-Day Walk.

My "hopeful" activity.

I don't want to meet these people doing the Breast Cancer Walk. I don't want to face *anyone* dealing with breast cancer, people who have lost mothers, daughters, *aunts*.

Been there. Done that. Don't need any more.

2

The bus made a wide circle at North Point. When it stopped, Emmy sat in stony silence. She was still pissed off that she had to be there, had to get off the bus, had to go meet a bunch of strangers—*had* to walk *seven miles*.

Most of the passengers departed, then a few got on, but Emmy sat, watching, wondering if she would get off, too.

At last, grabbing the Blowfish, she ran to the door and quickly jumped down to the concrete. She strode across Van Ness Avenue, shivering in the light morning breeze. Below her, fog covered the cold, gray waters of San Francisco Bay.

She glanced at the paper in her fingers. "Meet at Aquatic Park," it said, "at 8:00 AM for an easy flat 7 mile walk to Pac Bell Park and back."

Easy, she thought. *Yeah. Right.*

Unzipping the bulging mouth of the Blowfish, she poked the slip of paper inside, jamming it between Band-Aids, Neosporin, sunglasses, trail mix, sun screen, driver's license, Fast Pass, cash, and a banana. She knew it was overkill, but it was a comforting thought that when everything broke down she could bandage it, have a snack, and catch a bus home.

She forced the zipper closed, then lifted it to her hips and snapped the buckle into place. It felt heavy, especially with the two water bottles, one balanced on each hip.

Turning, she marched down the hill, peering through the fog at Aquatic Park.

It was hard to miss, with its circular pier enclosing a little pocket of the Bay. Above it, the Maritime Museum, looking ship-shape, faced outward. A beach ran fifty yards long below a wide, curving sidewalk, with two sets of bleachers, one on each side of the Museum.

A few people were gathered on the north bleachers. She swallowed hard and trotted up the steps.

A man who appeared to be in his mid-forties turned to face her. Although he was a little husky, his legs were all muscle. He wore blue running shorts and a Breast Cancer 3-Day shirt from the 2000 Walk. A blue bandanna was tied around his reddish hair like a doo rag, with a bright yellow star turned out in the very center. A pair of wire rimmed glasses framed his green eyes. Although his face was a little timeworn, it was clean-shaven and far from ugly.

"Looking for the Training Walk?" he asked.

"Yeah." She nodded.

He extended his hand. "David Cook," he said. He had a firm, reassuring grip. "I'm the Training Walk Leader. The sign-in sheet's over there by the backpack. Go ahead and get loosened up."

As she sauntered over to the sign-in sheet, she passed another man of around forty, lean, with horn-rimmed glasses and a silly grin. He wore a San Francisco Giants baseball cap and also a shirt from the 2000 Walk. Two girls stretched together a couple of rows up and a Chinese girl stood alone at the end, stretching her legs. The sheet had a lot of small print followed by a numbered grid with a few names already filled in: Kat Chen and Tom O'Laughlin, presumably the Chinese girl and funny guy.

She printed her name, but the next space was for her Walker Number. She closed her eyes and squeezed the pen tight. *Geez!*! It was the only thing she didn't pack!

Stupid! Stupid! Stupid!

"I'm sorry," she said, turning back to David. "I don't have my Walker Number with me."

"Don't worry about it today." He smiled at her. "It's a good idea to have it memorized."

Of course, that's what they said at the 3-Day office—and she forgot! She quickly scrawled in her signature.

The goofy guy—Tom she was certain—turned to her. "You'd better read that," he said. "You might be signing your life away."

The Chinese girl—Kat —laughed.

"He means you *are* signing your life away," she said. There was no trace of an accent. "It's a Waiver of Liability. No matter what happens on the training walk, you can't sue Avon or Pallotta TeamWorks."

"Or him," Tom added, pointing at David.

"That's right," David replied as he bent over to stretch. "I'm *completely* innocent."

Tom guffawed. "Yeah, he's innocent like pigs fly."

"Or men are faithful," Kat countered, grinning.

In spite of herself, Emmy smiled. She dropped the clipboard and found a place to stretch. No one else had their fanny packs on, so she dropped the Blowfish on the bench.

Kat moved closer. She had a round, brown face and large bright eyes, but there was nothing round about her body. It was lean and tight. She wore red Spandex shorts and a loose sleeveless tee shirt with a black sports bra underneath. She wore her long, black hair in a pony tail, poking through the back of a Raiders baseball cap.

Glancing at Emmy sideways, she grinned.

"I'll tell you my name, but only if you promise not to say 'Gesundheit' or 'God Bless you.'"

It took Emmy just a second to realize it was a joke. *Kat Chen. Gesundheit.* Emmy grinned.

"Sure."

"Kat Chen."

Both of the guys sneezed her name and the two girls above them convulsed in laughter. Kat laughed, too, as she stepped up to Tom and punched him on the shoulder. Grabbing his arm, he fell back laughing.

"Geez, Kat, you bruised my arm! I'm gonna sue!"

"You already signed the Waiver!" she cried out.

Emmy laughed with them, both amazed and happy at how much she liked these people. It relaxed her. It made walking seven miles seem more possible.

Kat turned back to her, still grinning.

"Emmy," she said quickly, holding out her hand.

Kat shook it energetically.

"I'm the crazy Chinese girl in this outfit." Nodding behind her, she added, "Bozo here is Tom. The girls are Joy and Ellen." From above, they waved to Emmy.

As they spoke, more people arrived. Some went directly to sign-in, others were pointed there by David.

"I take it you all know each other?"

"We met last spring when David started leading training walks," Kat explained as they stretched. "At first, we hated it—his routes are fast—and crazy with hills—but if you stick with it, you get a nice fat reward at the end."

"What's that?"

"An easy 3-Day. Breeze through the Walk." She giggled. "Hit all the port-o-potties before lines form. Get the best bananas. First ones in the showers, first ones in the chow lines, first ones in bed." She turned her head back to Tom. "*Not* the first ones to get to sleep!"

Laughing, Tom shook his head. He strolled over to them. "Look," he said, "I can't help it if the girls don't like Robin Williams routines at bed time."

A woman with short, red hair dropped the clipboard and it clattered to the concrete. She wore brown sweat pants and a brown top and her eyes flashed as she turned. "Geez, Tom!" she cried. "You pull that this year and I'll personally kick your butt up Hell Hill."

Tom laughed raucously, clapping his hands and throwing back his head.

"Hell Hill?" The question was out of Emmy's mouth before she could stop it.

"Day Two," Kat answered. "Sea level to Ridgeline."

Emmy stood rigid.

"Ridgeline? The Peninsula Ridgeline?"

The redhead nodded. "Twelve hundred foot elevation gain spread out over a measly three miles. Kicks everybody's butt. Not us."

Geez! It wasn't a hill—it was a mountain. Emmy knew she couldn't do it. Could she? Maybe if she trained with these guys... Maybe they could help her. In a flash, she knew it. She would have to train with them. She knew it in the pit of her churning stomach.

"I'm Emmy." She offered her hand to the redhead.

"Marianne. Welcome aboard." She smiled. It was a beautiful smile and it warmed Emmy clear through. It was weird to feel so good and she wasn't sure how to process it. She managed to return a shy smile.

"Listen up!" David called out. He picked up his backpack and clipboard, strolled back to the entry, and turned to face the crowd. "Welcome to Team Aquatic Park. It's now eight o'clock and this Training Walk is officially closed."

A girl ran up the stairs and signed the sheet as he held it up. She looked really young—too young really. The minimum age to participate was eighteen, so Emmy just qualified, but this girl looked about fourteen. David watched her from the corner of his eye, but didn't say anything until she finished.

"Today, we're doing our seven mile flat walk. Who needs a map?" A number of people held up their hands and he passed out a stack of papers. Emmy took one when it came around.* It was a simple route, highlighted with red arrows, straight along the wharf to Pac Bell Park and back. She folded it up and stuffed it into the Blowfish.

"We have two fifteen minute breaks, both at Embarcadero Four. That's about five minutes for the bathroom and ten minutes to stretch." Emmy was really looking forward to that first bathroom break. "When we get back, we'll stretch to cool down. By the way, we're starting our hill training next weekend."

Kat's groan echoed the pain in Emmy's stomach.

Hills already?

"If you haven't trained with us before, we work the hills pretty hard, so be prepared."

She felt sick. Now, she'd have to start walking up hills. She hated it, but she really wanted to train with Kat and the others. And, if she made it far enough, she'd eventually have to face "Hell Hill."

---

* See Map on Page 317.

Damn!

It was quiet, so she looked up at David Cook. He stood, resting his hands on his hips, peering out at them, waiting for the last rustles to die away before he raised his voice.

"Nothing is more important to me than your safety, so listen closely to the rules. We stop at every red light. I don't care if the nearest car is five miles away, we wait till it turns green before we go. Always look both ways before you step off *any* curb. Never walk in the street and always move through intersections with alacrity."

"I have a question!" It was Tom, holding up his hand. David stared at him, waiting. "Uh, which one is Alacrity? I don't think I've met her yet."

There was a tittering of laughter, then booing and groaning as Tom leaned against the rail, laughing at his own joke and holding his hands up as if to ward off any flying debris. David shook his head sadly and smiled at them.

"Beware of idiots," he said. Laughter erupted. There was some applause and Kat blew a shrill whistle in Emmy's ear.

David grinned at Tom as the chuckling died away.

"As we walk along the Embarcadero, try not to walk more than three abreast. Be courteous to other pedestrians because we'll be going through a lot of people. If you need to pass someone on the sidewalk, please call out ,'On your right!' or 'On your left!' as you approach them.

"As you walk along the sidewalk, be alert for broken glass, cracks, or other hazards—point them out to those behind you. If anyone feels distress, for any reason, please speak up. I can't fix something if I don't know it's broken.

"You must carry your health insurance card, a drivers' license or other proof of identity, along with your name, home address, phone number, blood type and emergency contacts."

Damn! She'd left her insurance card at home and didn't have contact information with her. She tried to look innocent, but when she glanced around no one seemed to care.

"No earbuds or headphones are allowed and neither are cell phones. If you brought one, keep it turned off except on breaks. I assume that everyone has an adequate supply of water and Gatorade. Use them. You must hydrate regularly."

She had plenty of water, but hated Gatorade. If there was any one of his instructions to ignore, that was it.

"If you get hungry, eat. If you run out of water or Gatorade, I always carry extra. Don't be afraid to ask. And always remember the 3-Day safety motto: 'Stay Alert, Stay Alive.'" Kat and Marianne whispered the words along with him. The safety motto was splattered on everything. It was hard to forget.

"As usual, we'll start out at three miles an hour. We'll accelerate to three-point-five. That's our cruising speed. But sometimes we'll burst to four, so stay alert."

Four miles an hour! Emmy gaped, gazing around her. A few women in the bleachers looked amazed, too, but everybody else just nodded like it was the norm.

"Does anyone have any questions?"

Yes, Emmy thought, *I'm filled with questions, but I'm not about to ask them now*. He waited for a few seconds, then nodded. "All right then. Let's move out."

He shouldered his backpack as they buckled on their fanny packs. This was it. She wasn't ready. *Please, don't let me wimp out half-way*. Her fingers fumbled at the belt and she just got it buckled as David trotted down the steps and strode up the sidewalk toward Pier 39. Tom stepped up beside him, with Kat and Marianne behind.

Emmy fell in toward the back. She'd been walking at about three miles an hour at lunch, so the beginning pace was comfortable. Two women stepped up beside her, one older and the other in her early twenties.

"Hey there," the older woman said. "I'm Karen and this is my daughter, Rhonda." The girl waved.

"Emmy," she answered.

"Where are you from?" Karen asked.

"Pleasanton—originally," she answered, "but I live in the Richmond District now. What about you guys?"

"We're from Fremont."

"Fremont? Geez, that's a long way!"

Rhonda chuckled. "I know, but the drive is worth it. It's the best training you can get."

More proof that she had to train with David. She had to stay with this group. She glanced at Rhonda.

"How come you guys are in the 3-Day?"

Rhonda stared into space for a moment.

"Mom's a two-time survivor."

"Last time, I had to get a mastectomy." Karen said.

"She's in remission seven years now," Rhonda added quickly. "What about you?"

Emmy gasped for air. Amy had to have a mastectomy her second time around, too. She opened her mouth, but all she could say was, "My aunt." Her voice cracked.

"Sorry," Rhonda said.

Suddenly, everyone was walking faster. Nodding at Emmy, Karen and Rhonda moved away. Surrounded by street vendors and tourists, Emmy threaded her way alone along the wharf. Half an hour ago, that would have made her happy, but now she wanted to walk with her new friends.

As she rounded Pier 39, the street curved south to become the Embarcadero and she was into her daily walk route. Short of breath, she stopped to drink water. She really wished she could walk faster. She had to lose more weight. She'd been so happy to lose six pounds this month, but if she kept walking and ate nothing but rabbit food, she could lose a lot more, especially when she started on hills.

There was no question now. She *really* had to pee!

She *had* to walk faster now. No choice. At least the fog had lifted and it was sunny. As she approached Embarcadero Four, the light turned red. *Damn!* She jogged in place and then sprinted across when it turned green. Speeding behind the fountain at Justin Herman Plaza, she ran up the steps up to the Lobby Level at E4 and straight to the bathroom. She knew right where it was because her job was at Markham Graphics was on the tenth floor of E2.

There was a steady stream in and out of the bathroom, so she only had to wait a minute before rushing inside.

One thing she had learned from depression was that something as simple as taking a pee can bring incredible joy. She shivered as relief washed over her. Now she could tell Barb that she'd had one moment of undiluted happiness.

She washed up and headed back out to the patio. Leaning on the railing above the burbling fountain, she stretched her right hamstring and gasped—that last burst of speed to reach the bathroom had really tightened it up.

David stepped up to her. "How you doing?"

"Good," she answered. "It's a little fast for me."

His smile was reassuring. "Don't worry. Just keep at it and you'll get your speed."

If only, she thought. *If only...*

Back downstairs, they crossed the Embarcadero and walked along the Bay toward Pac Bell Park. The Bay Bridge was high above them, towering like a skyscraper. It was gray and black, ugly compared to the Golden Gate, but so huge it was impressive just being itself. She walked as fast as she could to keep up; restaurants and sailboats streamed by and soon she approached the ballpark. David and Kat rounded the statue of Willie Mays and headed back. Up and down the line, they high fived those still on the way. Kat gave Emmy a big smile as they slapped hands and it really felt good.

Emmy wanted nothing more than to walk with her.

It started as an ache, but it built fast and she knew that she had to be up alongside Kat. She would have to work hard to get there. Walk—and lose more weight. Walk hills. Get faster. It felt like maybe she *wanted* this now. Maybe Barb and Tina were right. Maybe she *needed* to do this.

As she rounded the statue, David and the others picked up speed. She tried to go faster, but just couldn't. In fact, she fell further behind with each step and it hurt more and more and not just in her muscles. She was alone again and she couldn't stand it. It hurt so much she just wanted to stop and cry.

Wants aside, she wouldn't allow herself to cry. Not again. Not since the night she chugged a bottle of pills and lived to tell about it.

It was hard to lift each leg up the stairs at E4. At the top, she saw that the break was almost over. She went to the bathroom and when she got out, David and the others were gone. Leaning against the rail, she joined the other stragglers to stretch.

She felt so tired. She knew she couldn't go on.

Her Fast Pass was in the Blowfish and there was a cable car just a block away by the Hyatt Regency. She could be at Ross's apartment in twenty minutes. A hot bath. A cold Tsingtao. Maybe some cuddling.

It was a nice fantasy, but the others headed for the stairs to finish the walk. What would David and Kat think if she bailed? The safety lecture. *Geez!* Did David wait for everyone to return?

The last woman was just heading down the stairs.

"Excuse me!" Emmy called out. "Do they wait for us to get back?"

The woman stopped and smiled. "Sometimes. If you're not coming back, I can pass it along."

This was it. Now or never. She had to decide. Did she really want to do this? Did she want to be up front with Kat? Yes. She had to finish. *Damn it!* She had to go. She had to do this whole damn Walk and not just because Tina wanted her to or because she needed to lose the weight. She had to do it for herself. She had to do this whole damn thing for herself.

"No," she answered. "I'll finish."

Straightening up, she shuffled to the stairway and hobbled down to the street. She waited at the light and when it turned green, she took off. To spite the pain, she forced herself to walk at her normal pace. The pain itself pissed her off. *I've got to get better! I've got to!*

One by one, she began to pass the other stragglers. She was

walking alone, but she was determined to finish. A mile. Pier 39. Two. Her mind blank, empty. And then, there was Aquatic Park. Slowing down, she approached the bleachers.

David and the others were still stretching, so she joined them. The second she stopped walking, the pain *really* hit, but she stretched and it warmed down her muscles. It didn't take away the pain, but it made it easier to bear.

One by one, the other walkers left, just as the final few stragglers came in—and there was the woman she had talked to at E4, smiling as she passed. David watched to make sure they all returned and Emmy felt a flush of joy that she'd finished. David really *did* care about them.

Finishing up, she grabbed the Blowfish and moved slowly and painfully toward the bus stop, but there was a part of her that was really, really happy. She had walked the whole seven miles—and did pretty good in the end. She was proud of herself.

Waiting for the bus, she saw David trekking up Van Ness, wearing his backpack and marching along as if he hadn't just completed a high tempo seven mile walk.

Geez! He must walk down in the morning and home at the end—wearing a heavy pack, no less.

Why?

The bus rolled up and she climbed in, settling into a seat near the back as they headed south down Van Ness. Four miles an hour was brutal. Why did they walk so fast?

Of course! At four miles an hour, it would only take five hours to walk twenty miles. That's why they did it! "First ones to the port-o-potties. First ones to the showers."

That's smart. Real smart!

When the bus rolled past Lombard Street, she saw David Cook still plugging along. She admired him so much. He moved swiftly up the street, walking alone, walking fast, and walking with a definite sense of purpose.

3

Training Journal of Emmy Wells

1/28	Sunday	7 Miles, Flat, Team Aquatic Park.
1/29	Monday	3 Miles, Embarcadero, Pier 39.

Tuesday, January 30

"The hills scare me to death. There's a terrible hill on Day Two, so I've got to practice. I've got to go up and down hills all the time. Nobody told me about hills."

Dr. Jenner pursed her lips. "Emmy," she said, "you live in San Francisco. You should be used to hills."

Emmy shook her head.

"That's why God invented cable cars."

Barb laughed. "I guess if you've got to do it, you'll have to figure out how."

Emmy closed her eyes. It was crushing. Just thinking about the hurt made her want to bail on the whole project. She could still get in a nice lunch before work. Maybe Tina was available? Or Joanna? *Wait a minute. What she said: 'If you've got to do it...'*

"Do I?" Emmy asked. Barb stared at her. "I mean, it's not like this is work or school. I'm only doing it because you asked me to. I won't get fired or flunked if I just quit."

Barb held her gaze, perhaps a little perplexed.

"Didn't you tell me just five minutes ago how much you wanted to walk with that Chinese girl?"

Emmy turned her head and stared out the window. *Why did I have to open my big mouth about Kat?* Coit Tower stood tall atop Telegraph Hill, not more than a mile away.

"Maybe that's just a fantasy," she said.

"I don't think so." Barb sat up in her chair. "I think it's a legitimate goal that you can accomplish. If you work hard. And you can work hard. Look at how far you've come already. You've been walking almost every day. You're losing weight. You feel better. Do you really want to give up how good you felt on Sunday?"

Always in a corner. Always in a corner.

"Emmy." She leaned forward and touched Emmy's arm, forcing her into eye contact. "Tell me you don't want to feel that good again. Tell me that wasn't the happiest you've felt in months."

Suddenly, Emmy's eyes welled up.

I will not cry. I will not allow myself to cry.

"I can't."

"Then you have to do it," Barb said.

Emmy sighed. There was no way out. She would just have to do the damned hills.

"I've got an idea," she replied, "but I don't like it. I've been walking on the Embarcadero before work. I can shift over to California Street and do Nob Hill."

She heard the little intake of breath as Barb gasped. "Isn't that a little big to start out with?"

"If I'm gonna do it, I'd may as well do it right. A hill's a hill. You know what they call that big hill on Day Two?" Barb shook her head. "Hell Hill."

A little smile tugged at the corner of Barb's mouth.

"How appropriate."

Even though Barb couldn't contain her smile, Emmy saw little wet glints in the corners of her eyes. *I wish I could figure her out. I know she cares about what happens to me—I just wish she'd take some Valium or something to mellow out.*

"Yeah. Just what I need, huh? More hell."

As she left the building, Emmy remembered again that blank space in her memory, that blackout. It hadn't come up.

What happened after she had seen Grace crying on the path?

4

Training Journal of Emmy Wells

2/4	Sunday	6 Miles, flat, Golden Gate Park.
2/5	Monday	Appx. 1/2 Mile? Solo, Nob Hill.
2/6	Tuesday	Appx. 3/4 Mile? Solo, Nob Hill.

Wednesday, February 7, 11:30 am

I can't believe this is my *4th* day on this damned hill. Last Friday, I only got a block and a half before I turned back. A block and a half! I hate myself for quitting, but I went back on Monday and made it a half-block farther to Grant Street—two blocks up the hill—and quit again. I added one more block yesterday—to Stockton. I swear I've never hurt more. The ache is total. It's who I am now. Utterly me. I hobbled around my classes all morning, but this is the day.

I'm gonna make it all the way to the Fairmont Hotel.

I hate this damned hill. I hate it. I hate it. But I've got to get it done. I've got to beat the son of a bitch. I've got to do it. Even though I don't want to do it. I don't want to go up this damned hill and sweat and ache. Worst of all, I *hate* myself for not wanting to do it. All I want in life right now is to sit with Tina at the London Wine Bar and attack a Cobb salad smothered in bacon and blue cheese.

But I can't.

I can't!

I've got to do this.

I've got to climb hills and walk farther and faster.

If I want to walk beside Kat—and I really want to walk beside Kat—I'll do it.

If it kills me.

5

She pushed through the door at Markham Graphics and hobbled to the bathroom with her gym bag. It hurt. Every step hurt, but she gritted her way through it.

Pain ripped through her back as she tugged her jeans down over her hips, then it tore back through her hamstrings and calves as she pulled on her shorts.

She dropped off her gym bag with Joanna, the receptionist, then turned to the elevator and wedged a bottle of water into the Minnow. She hated the Blowfish and didn't need it for short walks like this. Aside from Fast Pass, insurance card, and ID, the water was all she needed. She'd written her blood type and contact information on the back of a business card, so if she got heart palpitations, went into cardiac arrest, spazzed all over the sidewalk oozing drool, and expired, at least someone would know she had insurance and was Type A Positive.

She packed herself into the elevator with designer suits and dresses and they all gave her a wide berth. She smiled. Residual stink in her walking clothes.

Having a nice day, Mr. Armani? Smell this.

Out of the elevator at Street Level, she stopped at the side of the building to stretch and was done in two minutes. There was no time to waste. Dashing up Clay Street, she turned left at the Transamerica Pyramid and worked her way to California, then started up Nob Hill. It was amazing how easy the first block had become, but the second block tilted upward mercilessly.

The burn kicked in, but she felt strong enough to handle it. *Geez*, she thought ruefully, *I'm used to it now.* Pushing steadily, she reached Grant Street. She stopped on the corner by the Chinatown McDonalds. Her lungs pumped air and sweat filled the band of her baseball cap.

Glancing up the narrow, bricked street with little green dragons perched over the shops, she unzipped the Minnow and chugged water. The smell of oil and incense surrounded her. Looking up the hill, she thought she could even smell the sunshine that brightened the concrete before her. Even though she was sweating, a shiver passed through her.

I'm gonna make it. I know I'm gonna make it!

She started again, leaning into the slope. The sidewalk tilted up, only a foot in front of her nose. Step after step, she pushed herself up the block. It went on forever. Halfway up, she stopped and wiped away the sweat that ran into her eyes. It streamed down her arms and splatted on the sidewalk. Her legs trembled, but she started again, pushing harder until she stepped up onto the even concrete of Powell Street.

A cable car edged over the hill, heading down toward the Bay. Tourists laughed and the bell clanged merrily, but Emmy still had another block to go. She tingled. One more block. The slope didn't look as bad as the others. She *could* make it. She *would* make it. *It's time to beat this damned hill.*

Stepping forward, she worked her way up the last block. Pain shot from her hips to her back, but she forced her legs to move, one damn step after another, sucking air, blowing air, sucking in more. Sweat ran down her cheeks, neck and chest, but still she pushed on, up the last few steps to the very last step.

Top of the world.

She strode back and forth sucking air, then stopped. The entrance to the Fairmont, tall and stately, stood before her. She wanted to feel happy, but all she felt was relief. She just felt relieved. It was done. Done and over. Hobbling to the hotel, she placed both palms against the smooth, cool stone of the building.

It was over.

Over and done.

Pushing off against the building, she stretched her legs, warming down, loosening up the muscles. A cable car would be along any minute, so she hobbled over to California Street and stared up at the sweeping peaks of Grace Cathedral. There was no cable car.

Turning, she blew out a long breath and lifted off her baseball cap. It was soaked. She wrung it out and the sweat dribbled and splashed onto the sidewalk.

Down toward the Bay, she saw the tops of buildings on the waterfront. *The tops!* Her gaze traveled down the hill. The street was a mosaic of traffic—like some great river in a canyon of buildings.

At the very end, far below, lay the serene waters of San Francisco Bay.

6

Training Journal of Emmy Wells

2/7	Wed.	1 Mile, Solo, Nob Hill.
2/8	Thursday	Rest.
2/9	Friday	Rest.

Saturday, February 10, 6:35 am

I took Thursday and Friday off and barely managed to drag my ass to lunch each day, once with Tina and once with Ross. He asked me to spend last night at his place so he could give me a ride this morning and I'm thankful. I still hurt from Nob Hill and I'm totally exhausted, so I'm really grateful for the lift.

He's so tolerant of me, I can't quite believe it. I met him in the hall at work last November. He doesn't work for us—he's a copy writer with the Beckman agency and he was working with Marcy on a special project. I remember she laughed at something he said. I thought he was cute and smiled just as he looked up and saw me and that was sort of it.

At first, I thought he was a mirage or something, but he kept asking me out, even after he knew me. He's smart and funny. I like him, but I have no idea why he's stayed with me.

So here I am, with a ride and hopefully ready to walk again. It's eight miles today, my longest walk yet, but I need to build on Nob Hill while the work is fresh. I'm going to take a Motrin before we leave.

Maybe that'll help.

7

Ross shifted his Scoupe into second as the light changed at Lombard, then roared ahead down Van Ness toward Aquatic Park. Sitting across from him, Emmy felt strangely relaxed. Instead of nerves for her first hill walk with the team, she just felt tired and resigned to the ordeal. He pulled up to the curb and she picked up the Blowfish from the floor.

"Thanks for the ride." She leaned in for a quick kiss.

"Take it easy today," he answered, smiling.

"I will. We should be done by about ten forty-five."

"I'll be here."

She eased herself out, then turned and sauntered down to the concrete bleachers. She trudged up the steps, but there were only a few people there. She moved next to Kat so they could stretch together. From a lunge position, Kat looked at her sideways.

"Hey! Welcome back. Done any hills yet?"

"Yeah," Emmy answered.

"Where'd you go?" Tom asked.

"California Street. Downtown."

"Geez!" Kat cried. "You picked a whopper!"

"Hey, hey, hey!" It was a bellow coming from back at the entrance. "This *must* be the training walk!" Emmy looked back to see a muscular black guy wearing yellow Spandex and red Nikes. He grinned at everyone. "Michael Bay!" he announced, opening his arms wide. "To brighten your day!"

David grinned and pointed to the sign-in sheet. Walking toward the clipboard, Michael smiled and said Hi to everyone he passed. Most of the women watched his muscles ripple, even though it was rather obvious he was gay.

"Well," Tom muttered, his eyes twinkling, "this should be interesting."

Michael turned to stretch and David retrieved his backpack. He looked around for a moment, then put away the clipboard.

"Morning, all! Today we're doing an eight mile walk with two hills. Who needs a map?" Emmy took one and glanced at it.* She didn't recognize the first part of the route. "We're starting with Russian Hill," he said casually, "by way of Hyde Street."

---

* See Map on Page 319.

"Geez, David!" Kat scowled from her knee bend.

Damn. It must be a bad one.

Marianne grinned and that confirmed it.

"We'll follow it up with Telegraph Hill. Just two hills and we get 'em out of the way early. After that it's just a fun walk along the Embarcadero." His safety lecture was also more relaxed for this smaller group and once again there were no questions.

"All right then," he said, "Let's go."

He shouldered his backpack, jogged down the steps, and strode briskly down the sidewalk to the cable car turnaround. Kat moved up beside him, with Tom and Marianne falling in right behind. Emmy found a place in the middle and that was okay with her, better than at the end.

A middle-aged woman with short black hair and a strong nose fell into step beside her.

"Hey, there," she said. "Haven't seen you before."

"I just started training."

She laughed. "Honey, you picked a doozy to start with. You train any hills yet?"

Emmy nodded. "I did Nob Hill."

"I mean has anyone *trained* you how to do hills?"

"No, I guess not."

"I'll walk with you." She smiled. "Help you out."

"Thanks. I'm Emmy."

"Janet."

They headed up past the Buena Vista on Hyde, stopping at a red light at Bay Street. As they waited for it to change, Emmy raised her eyes to look up at the Hyde Street hill. It was similar to Nob Hill. Cable car rails ran down the middle of the street and it sloped at close to forty-five degrees for forever.

"Holy shit!" It was Michael Bay and he was right beside her. Turning his head, he stared at her with wide eyes. "Would you look at that bitch? Who dreams up this shit anyway?"

David turned to face Michael with a bright smile.

"I do," he replied. "It's just a little incline. Shouldn't give a big guy like you any trouble at all."

As he turned back to face the hill, Michael shielded his eyes and whispered, "Little incline?"

Up front, Joy and Ellen flexed their legs and Kat pushed herself up on her toes, bouncing in place. The light turned green, so they crossed together and started up the hill. All Emmy could see without craning her neck was the sidewalk in front of her nose, but Janet was on one side of her and Michael on the other.

Janet nodded. "Couple of pointers," she said. "Take smaller steps. When you stride on a hill, it puts stress on your Achilles. Also, try not to lean forward. Just keep an erect posture. Otherwise, you could hurt your back."

Emmy was amazed that she could even talk, let alone give advice, but she did what Janet said and it *did* help. Michael matched his steps to hers.

Turning her head slightly, she smiled at Janet.

"Thanks!" she panted.

After they had gone about fifty paces, Janet glanced over at them. "I gotta go," she said. "See you at the top."

Janet easily accelerated up the hill as Emmy worked to catch her breath. She and Michael glanced at each other and kept pushing. About two-thirds of the way up, she couldn't breathe anymore. Stopping, she gasped for air. Michael stopped, too, and they both drank water. Wiping sweat from his brow, he glanced at her fat.

"Damn, girl, you got some go."

She smiled. He was all muscle, but she had the go. That was pretty cool. When she had her breath back, they kept pushing. It hurt, but not as bad as Nob Hill. At the end of the block, the street was level, but on the other side it went up again.

Michael wiped more sweat from his brow and muttered, "Gotta get a sweat band." They drank again, then continued on. Fortunately, that block wasn't nearly as long—or as steep.

Straining, she heaved her way to the very top of the hill. Sweat rolled down the side of her face and over her neck. Her baseball cap was soaked again and she gasped for air.

David and the others stood together, laughing at some joke as if nothing out of the ordinary had just occurred. Most of them were still sweating, but no one looked tired and no one was gasping for breath.

"Would you look at that!" Michael whispered, pointing out across the Bay. From the top of Russian Hill, they saw the black Marin Headlands pushing up beyond the Golden Gate Bridge. Sausalito nestled against the eastern side, houses perched on the hillside all the way down to the colorful sailboats in the Bay. And there was Alcatraz, a white prison blooming from its wild green shore, and Angel Island.

She noticed cars queued up on the side streets and suddenly realized they were standing on Lombard at the corner of "the crookedest street in the world." The cars were waiting their turn to zig and zag down the loopy street from Russian Hill to North Beach.

"Good job," David said, strolling over to them. Taking Emmy's elbow, he walked them off to the side. "Part of the trick with hills is regular breathing. Find a rhythm that's comfortable. Steady intake through the nose. Count it out with every step, then let it out slowly through the mouth, same number of steps. Don't blow it out, let it out easy."

Emmy nodded. "Thanks."

"Don't forget to hydrate," he added, turning away.

"Sounds good," Michael agreed, reaching for a bottle. "I hope he knows what he's talking about."

"You can trust David," she answered, surprised by her own surety.

The route took them south through rolling hills. She wasn't familiar with Russian Hill, but it was nice. There were lots of trees, little corner stores and some pretty little houses.

They turned left and started east, over another small hill that wasn't too hard, then down into Chinatown and North Beach. They passed little Italian restaurants and bistros gleaming in bright sunshine, then crossed busy Columbus Avenue and started uphill again. It got steep fast and they cut around to begin a steeper climb.

It was Telegraph Hill.

As she labored steadily upwards, Emmy used David and Janet's advice. She found a natural rhythm to her breathing and set her pace to work with it. Small steps. Steady breathing. Keep erect. Her pace was slow, but it suited her, and although she fell behind, it didn't matter.

The street ended at a long concrete stairway that seriously hurt her shins as she tramped upward, ever upward. She stayed at her own pace, one foot in front of the other, and soon joined the others, breathing almost normally. They were not at the crest; she couldn't see Coit Tower looming above them.

Kat grinned and slapped her hand. She had no idea it could feel so good just to reach the top of a hill. And step by step, it began to add up. It got easier. The pain was her badge of honor.

Stretching, she felt the burn all the way down, but it was a good burn. Her muscles were getting stronger.

The last person topped out and they turned to work their way down the eastern side of the hill, down toward the Bay. They zig-zagged down a switchback, then David led them into a garden—a wide open space with houses on both sides clinging to the hill. Stairs ran down the side and a canopy of trees shaded lush flower gardens. It was beautiful.

Tom looked up into the trees and shook his head.

"No parrots today."

"What?"

"Wild parrots live here, at least part of the time."

At the end of the garden, an extremely long stairwell led down to Levi Plaza. Step by step, her shins ached with the pain of it, all the way down to the street.

During the break at E4, she wandered over to stretch with David. Michael joined them and asked for advice on how to stretch.

For a guy loaded with muscle, she thought, *he sure doesn't know much about walking.*

They continued on to Pac Bell Park, slapped hands around Willie Mays, and returned to E4 for a second break. Heading back to Aquatic Park, in the middle of the pack, Emmy worked on her speed. As hard as she tried to keep up with the lead walkers, she just couldn't do it. On the other hand, she was much faster than last time and felt good about that. She was getting better.

And she would get faster. She would keep losing weight. And she would do better on hills.

And some day, she knew, she would walk up front.

8

Training Journal of Emmy Wells

2/15	Thursday	1.5 Miles, Nob Hill.
2/16	Friday	3 Miles, Embarcadero, Pier 39.

Saturday, February 17, 7:05 am

Everything's different this morning. I had to wake Ross up so he could give me a ride and he's in an awful mood. How could he be pissed about getting up a half hour early? I'm grateful for the ride, but if it makes him mad, I'd rather just take the bus.

Today we're doing a ten mile walk—the longest so far. I can do it. I know I can, but it'll be a lot of work and I'm getting sick of hurting all the time. Tomorrow's another seven mile flat walk and I'm going, but I'll skip the eight mile hill walk on Monday—President's Day—because Ross and I are taking a day for ourselves. I'll just walk solo in the morning.

9

The silence in the car felt downright oppressive. Ross stared straight ahead all the way down to Aquatic Park. He pulled up to the curb and she leaned over to touch his hand.

"Thanks, Ross. I'm really sorry it's early, but the more we walk, the earlier it's gonna get."

He sighed. "I know. Sorry I'm all crabby. I'm not very good with mornings."

"I can take the bus from home. It's not a big deal."

"No," he answered quickly, smiling for the first time. "I'll get used to it. I like having you stay with me."

She kissed him, not quick and easy, but something to let him know just how much it meant to her.

"We should be done by eleven."

She hustled across the lawn to the bleachers and joined Kat down at the rail. Tom smiled at her as he stretched, then he stopped, glancing at her quizzically.

"I'm sorry, I forgot your name."

"Emmy," Kat said. "Don't you ever pay attention?"

"Not 'til I see somebody the third or fourth time. You know how it is, Kat: people come, people go."

"Yeah," she sighed. "Not everybody sticks."

Emmy looked directly into Tom's eyes.

"I'm here to stay."

"Sorry," he repeated. "Sometimes I'm an idiot."

Marianne strolled over. "Sometimes?"

Laughter peeled around them as Tom grinned at her.

"Good morning!" Michael called out as he strutted over to them. "What kind of wicked hills we got today?"

Marianne grinned. "We got a couple little inclines and then the Big Kahuna. Pacific."

It didn't sound familiar. Emmy looked up. "Pacific?"

"Pacific Street hill," Kat explained. "Leave it to David to add some hill toward the end, just to put the cherry on top."

"Oh, it's not a bad hill," Marianne said. "It's just where it comes. You think you're home free and then there's this little monster. Eats you alive."

Emmy felt her stomach flip. *Just what I need—a little monster at the end.*

Story of my life.

"Ten miles," Janet said. "Half-way to the average."

Emmy turned to her. "Average?"

"Each day's a different mileage," Marianne said. "Last year, Day One was twenty-three and a half miles. Day Two was sixteen—Hell Hill. The third day was a little over twenty."

Tom nodded at Emmy. "Don't worry, we train twenty-three miles a couple times before the 3-Day. David has it all worked out."

Michael grinned. "We're training with the Marquis de Sade—in New Balance shoes!"

"I notice you came back," Marianne smirked.

"Maybe I'm a sub-dom. Is that it? A sub-dom?"

Tom tilted his head back, laughing. "A sub!" he called out. "You're a sub—David's the dom!" Joy and Ellen giggled hysterically and everyone laughed. Michael winked at Tom to show he was only joking.

"Okay, everybody!" David called out. "Listen up." He strolled to his briefing spot holding up the clipboard. "It's seven-thirty and this training walk is closed."

The same young girl as before quickly ran up to him and signed in as he held the clipboard for her. Looking at the group, he rolled his eyes in mock exasperation. Smiling, she faded back into the group.

"Today we're doing a ten mile hill walk—the northern route for a change of pace. Who needs a map?"

Emmy took one.*

It looked like an awfully long route, but it was hard for her to estimate mileage when the lines squiggled all over the page. "We begin with a nice easy walk along the shore to the Golden Gate Bridge Toll Plaza, where we'll take our first break. Then, we'll head up through the Presidio on a nice *long incline*. Pace yourselves. We end up at Mountain Lake, where we'll take our second break, then we take the Pacific Street hill and head home."

When he reached the end of the safety lecture, Tom, Kat, and Marianne joined him in the safety motto:

"Stay Alert, Stay Alive."

As they started out, Emmy positioned herself near the front of the group. It was the first time, but that's where she wanted to be and she felt ready to try it out. They started out slow, joining in the flow of people heading up into Fort Mason, down under the tall trees through the grassy lawn toward the Marina.

The cute little girl that always signed in late moved up beside her. "Hi," she said. "I'm Juliette."

See Map on Page 321.

"Emmy."

Juliette's long hair was dun blond and her blue eyes brightly sparkled. Her tee shirt bore the logo of the American Cancer Society and it was covered in signatures.

"You mind if I ask how old you are?"

Juliette laughed. "Don't feel bad. I'm eighteen."

Emmy grinned. "Me, too. You've graduated?"

"Yeah. Freshman at SF State. You?"

"Art Institute."

When Emmy glanced at her shirt, Juliette smiled sadly.

"The first day I signed up," she said, "I had my mom and my aunt sign this. They're both survivors. Then all my friends wanted to sign it and it kind of snowballed."

Her mother and her aunt. Geez.

"At least they're survivors."

"I hate that word," Juliette answered. Emmy glanced sharply at her. "No one should have to go through that," she explained. "I sat up with my mom every night during the chemo. She was sick all the time. We didn't think she'd survive the damn drugs. It was horrible."

Emmy didn't have an answer for that, but "survivor" wasn't a bad word to her.

"At least she's alive," she replied. It came out very harsh and she wanted to take it back. Juliette glanced at her as they hustled along, then nodded her head. They walked in silence, passing yachts anchored next to the Marina Green and Emmy tried not to think about Amy.

Then David picked up the speed and all she could think about was breathing. She was comfortable at three and a half mph now. It felt good. She just couldn't talk.

They left the Marina behind and took a little path out along the Bay. To the west, the ruddy struts of the Golden Gate Bridge rose into the milky sky. She'd never seen it from underneath, but it was easy to pick out Fort Point in the distance. When they were almost there, David led them up a little road that curved up into the Presidio. *A little incline. Yeah.*

As she ascended, Emmy felt her legs tighten up, but it wasn't long until they marched into the parking lot that abutted the south side of the Golden Gate Bridge.

After a short bathroom break, they headed back out and continued up a very long hill into the Presidio, into a forest of pine and eucalyptus. If the whole thing hadn't gone steadily uphill, she might have enjoyed it, but the strain on her legs and hips grew until the pain was intense. Her left leg cramped, a sharp pain that bit into her calf.

She shook it, stretching the muscle with each step, but it was killing her. She fell back.

Eventually, when she topped out, the leaders had moved on, except for Juliette, who seemed to be keeping track of her. She was coated in sweat, gasping for air in spite of her pacing. Worst of all, she felt light-headed and dizzy.

Walking down a little street past the gigantic abandoned Marine Hospital, she felt weaker and weaker and fell steadily behind. *What's wrong with me?* They were about seven miles in—she'd done that much before without fainting away like a baby.

As she stepped through the gate that separated the Presidio from the City, she stumbled and felt herself enveloped in Juliette's arms. They walked together, Juliette helping her as they crossed Park Presidio. On the other side, there was a little path that led over a tiny hill. It was only about twenty feet long and fifteen feet high, yet Emmy could barely get up it. The world reeled around her and she sucked in air faster than she could process it.

At the top, Juliette called out, "David! Something's wrong with Emmy!" As they struggled down the slope, the world tilted and shifted, as if everything was out of alignment.

"Bring her here!" David called back. He and Juliette sat her down on the bench of a picnic table. He took off her soaked baseball cap and she realized she was coated in sweat.

Dizziness. Such dizziness. It won't let go.

Yanking both of her bottles from the Blowfish, David dropped them on the grass.

"Where's your Gatorade?" he asked.

Blowing out a deep breath, she worked to steady herself. She shook her head, loopy and candid. "Can't drink it," she gasped. "Vile." He reached for his backpack and pulled out a large bottle of red liquid.

Gatorade.

"I don't care if it's vile," he said. "You're dehydrated and water isn't going to help. You need this." Twisting off the cap, he held the bottle up to her mouth. "Drink!"

His command forced her to open up. As he carefully poured, she eagerly gulped it down, hardly tasting it, suddenly hungry for every drop. Her hands gradually took control of the bottle and she drank continuously.

Chuckling, he picked up one of her water bottles and poured out half of the water. She pulled the Gatorade away from her mouth to protest, but just gasped. He poured Gatorade into her water bottle until it was full.

"It'll help the taste if it's mixed with water, but you have to drink it. I'm *not* going to lose anybody from *dehydration*. Drink up."

He handed it back to her and she tilted it to her lips. The water *did* temper the taste. He watched her carefully as she drank. After a couple of gulps, she pulled it away from her mouth, but he waved his finger at her to keep drinking. When she was about to burst, he relented.

"Finish it all before we leave," he said. He poured out half the water in her other bottle and filled it up with more Gatorade. As she sipped in silence, he lifted his head and looked her in the eye.

"I haven't met anybody yet who likes the taste, but you have to drink it. You're an athlete now and when your muscles work hard and you sweat that much, you're not just losing water, you're losing sodium and vitamins and minerals that your body needs for a walk like this. I don't want to see you on another training walk unless you have at least one bottle of Gatorade. Mix it with water, I don't care, but always bring it."

As he spoke, she drank the last of the bottle. It was amazing how much better she felt. Her fingers weren't trembling, she was fully cooled down, and now fully back in reality.

Stupid! So incredibly stupid! Why didn't I drink at the Toll Plaza or while I was walking? It's so basic that the 3-Day people chant it like a rain dance:

"Hydrate! Hydrate! Hydrate!"

"Are we clear on that point?" he asked, looking into her eyes. A little smile tugged at the corner of his mouth.

He won't let this go until I agree.

She nodded. "Thanks, David."

Standing up, he looked around at the group.

"What's our mantra for the day?"

Marianne lifted her bottle of Gatorade. "Hydrate!" Around the group, one bottle after another was lifted in a toast and each voice called out, "Hydrate! Hydrate! Hydrate!"

Before he turned away, David glanced back down at her.

"Don't forget to pee."

It was unnecessary advice. She went to the restroom, ate her banana and a handful of trail mix, then stretched sheepishly with the others. She sat down in the grass and stretched out her legs. Leaning toward her left knee, she saw Mountain Lake for the first time. An Asian family stood tossing bread into the water as ducks dipped their heads to fish it out. An elderly couple sat on a bench.

It was peaceful, but she had no time to enjoy it.

They walked along the lake, then headed up a hill behind the driving range of the Presidio Golf Course under a leafy canopy. Michael walked beside her, almost like he was looking out for her. *His turn*, she thought ruefully. They passed by the clubhouse, then down a nice gentle path until they crossed over to Pacific Street.

It began as an alley next to the wall separating the City from the Presidio and as it became a street it was hard to miss the damned hill. Maybe Marianne had been right and it was small, but it sure looked like a whopper to Emmy.

And sure enough, it went on forever. The others attacked it, some with gleeful masochism, others with a blend of will and resignation, but she was happy to take her time, watching her breathing and pacing herself. Michael paced her, too. Twice, she stopped to drink from her spiked water and when she finally joined the others at the top, she was just happy it was over. She'd ground it out and survived.

Walking past the palatial homes of Presidio Heights, she slowed down again, falling toward the back. Maybe it was a dream that she could ever earn a space at the front. She did okay at the beginning but now she was back at the end.

Every step was like a little death, but every step brought her closer to home. All she could think about was a nice, hot bath and a Tsingtao. They stopped on Van Ness at the benches for warmdown stretching.

In spite of her dehydration, she began to feel okay again. Sure, her muscles ached, but she knew she would be alright—and in more ways than one. She'd found a group of people that cared about each other and looked after each other. She felt like she was a part of something much bigger than herself.

"Hey, Emmy," Kat said. "Don't look now but I think some pervert is ogling you."

She turned to face the street. The Scoupe was parked at the curb and Ross sat on the hood, his arms crossed casually, admiring her.

"That's okay. The pervert is my boyfriend."

"Oh," Kat said, glancing back at him. "He's cute."

10

Training Journal of Emmy Wells

2/18	Sunday	7 Miles Flat, Team Aquatic Park
2/19	Monday	5 Miles Flat, Solo, Cliff House.

Monday, February 19

Sitting on the sofa, Emmy crossed her left leg over her right and lifted her foot until she could study the bottom of it. There—right at the apex of the ball—was a little red spot.

On her morning walk, she had felt it start to burn, so she slowed down and that was probably all that kept it from turning into a big, nasty blister. Pulling out a tube of Neosporin, she slathered it good, bandaged it, then ran gauze all around the foot.

She had walked five miles that morning, down to Golden Gate Park, out to the Cliff House and back. There was even a little hill. Back before she met Ross, she used to take the bus to Cliff House to sketch people. It was built in the late 1800's on the side of a little cliff over the ocean. There was a restaurant in the main building and, off to the right, a smaller building with a hot dog stand. There was a narrow concrete stairway between that led to a patio with a sea wall, a Camera Obscura, and a museum of mechanical toys.

A horn blasted twice. It was Ross. She took a second to grab her carryall, waved goodbye to her roommate, Angie, and flew down the stairs. The Scoupe was double parked on 23rd Avenue, in front of the apartment. She dropped the carryall in the backseat and eased into the passenger bucket.

"Hey, Ross! How are you?"

"Good," he smiled, kissing her quickly. "Got a lot of writing done this morning. It's a good day."

They drove down along Golden Gate Park—the same route she had walked in the morning, except at Ocean Beach Ross turned south down the Peninsula.

He was quiet, but then he was always quiet. He had been trying to get some of his short stories published with no luck. Emmy thought he was pretty good. His mind was always in the clouds thinking about people that only existed in his head.

Not that I mind, she thought. *I like the quiet, too.*

In fact, she wouldn't want a boyfriend who chattered all the time, asking questions she didn't want to answer and getting into her personal life. There were some things she just didn't want to talk about. The first night they spent together, she had told him that her parents were divorced, but not about her father screwing his secretary or the midnight screaming fight or about her brother Dean's using her face as a punching bag. Although she told him about her wonderful sisters, Grace and Jill, she left out her insane mother. And her attempted suicide. And her ongoing therapy. And she definitely didn't tell him *anything* about Amy. The last thing she needed was sympathy.

Cold, foamy breakers rolled in to the beach. People strolled along, some throwing sticks for their dogs, some jogging. A few people stretched out on the sand, watching the endless sea.

Passing Lake Merced, they headed up into the heights on Skyline Boulevard. The ocean fell away as they rose higher and higher along the Peninsula Ridgeline. She knew that any of this terrain might be part of Day Two—from the Bay all the way to the top—Hell Hill. Cutting over to the Pacific Coast Highway, they came out on the very top of the crest that ran all the way south along the San Andreas Fault. It was an almost impossible drop to the ocean!

It seemed impossible, but it wasn't.

All the hills they walked on any given weekend probably totaled up to this one killer hill. She did that every weekend now and it didn't scare her any more.

I can do it, she thought with satisfaction.

Points to Barb on that.

They plummeted down the highway toward Pacifica. It was a scary height, but it was nothing compared to the prospect of raising nineteen hundred dollars.

She'd been putting it off, but a day of reckoning was coming. It sounded easy. All she had to do was ask for money. It must be easy for some people, but it scared her to death. And it wasn't just nerves. Her donation letter sucked. She'd tried to use the 3-Day samples, but it just sounded phony coming from her.

Ross had volunteered to help, but if the letter didn't sound like her now, she could only imagine the spin a professional ad man would put on it. Did they really need to strain a happy friendship based on nothing more than sex and comfort? She liked Ross. She was happy with the way things were. She'd rather not have him tied up in something so personal as this donation letter.

Excuses. The real reason she was putting it off was that she didn't want to think about Amy. To write her letter, to ask for money from the people who mattered, she'd have to talk about Amy. And, if she was honest with herself, she couldn't bring herself to do it. Hell, Barb had worked that ground pretty hard and all she ever got was Emmy's stony silence. No, she couldn't talk about it. Maybe ever.

So, her letter consisted of two words:

"Remember Amy..."

...and there it remained.

Emmy shook herself. She had to stay focused on the good stuff: walking and losing weight. The day of financial reckoning would come, but she didn't have to face it today. There were still five months left before the Walk. She'd figure it out somehow.

They zigged and zagged up through a little forest inland from Pedro Point and came out on the cliffs over the ocean. The Scoupe slowed. Ross pulled into a scenic overlook and parked. Leaning across the console, she kissed him, but the gear shift hurt, so she settled back in her seat and held his hand.

The sea stretched out before them so far that the curvature of the earth gently humped the ocean up in the distance. Gulls flew up to the cliffs and hung in front of the Scoupe, then darted away. The sky was a deep, dark blue and the salty air chilly. She turned her head to look at Ross and he smiled back at her, his eyes glinting in the afternoon sun.

He looked like he wanted to say something, but thankfully he didn't.

It was twilight as they approached Moss Beach. There was a restaurant perched on the cliffs overlooking the ocean, with a great salmon dish and a wonderful Merlot. Sitting at a table looking out to sea, moonlight glittering on the waves, she felt completely at peace.

Ross turned to her, looking a little shy.

"I was wondering—" he said. "What would you think... about moving in together?"

She stared at him stupidly, then laughed.

"Seriously?"

He nodded, smiling shyly. "We spend the weekends together anyway and quite a few weeknights. We'd save a lot of money. It would be a sure way of finding out if we're really compatible."

She stared at him. He was perfectly serious. She smiled to soften her answer.

"I'm not sure I want to know that." He squinted at her, but didn't say anything. She peered across the table. "You've given this some thought."

"Yes."

She was shocked. They hadn't known each other very long. It was a minefield. To begin with, he was four years older than her. *I haven't even told Mom about us.* She would have to soften up her mom long before she introduced him. She'd have to give Angie plenty of notice. She was totally unprepared for this!

He waited until she had to speak up.

"I need some time," she answered.

"Okay," he replied. His lips quirked into a smile. "At least it's not a no."

"It'll have to wait until after the 3-Day," she said.

Shit! If they moved in together, it would change everything! What if they *weren't* really compatible? And there was another thing that bothered her—why didn't he call at Christmas when he was in L.A.?

An entire week and not one word. She had to know.

"How come you didn't call? Over the holidays?"

His eyes clouded over. Maybe it was the wrong time to ask. He looked away and it scared her. *Maybe he has a girlfriend back home.* She couldn't breathe waiting for an answer.

Shifting in his chair, he stared out at the ocean.

"I wanted to," he answered quietly, "but things are... messy at home right now. I didn't want to dump it all on you at Christmas. If I'd called, I would have—and I didn't want to. That's all."

He turned his head to look at her. His eyes glistened in the light and she knew she'd touched a place that was very tender.

"What's wrong?"

He sighed. Was it wrong for her to ask? Was she forcing him to talk when he didn't want to? It seemed unfair and she hated herself for it. *I have secrets, too.*

"You know my dad died," he whispered.

"Yes," she answered, "a few years ago, right?"

"Yeah. He was a TV writer. Mostly cop dramas. Put in long hours, smoked like a chimney. In the old days, the writers sat around a table and just threw ideas at each other till they had a show. Most of them smoked. Anyway, my dad got lung cancer."

He stopped, his breath shallow. And suddenly she knew that their secrets were the same.

She nodded.

"It was long... hard. He passed in '96. They both used to drink a lot, but after he died, Mom lived on bourbon.

"We moved to smaller and smaller houses till Kath and I were both gone. Now she's in a little bungalow in Burbank. Before Christmas, she got fired and... well, like I said, it's messy. We're helping her out with money, but Kath's taken the brunt of trying to sober her up and get her back on her feet." He blew out a breath. "See why I didn't want to ruin your Christmas?"

"I'm sorry. I didn't know."

"Well, see, I managed to ruin things anyway."

"No!" She wrapped her hand around his head and caressed him. "I'm glad you told me." Even though it was terrible about his mom, it was good to know his family was as messed up as hers. Maybe that was unfair.

Maybe all families are messed up.

Maybe mine isn't so bad.

And even if her family *was* screwed up, at least they still had each other. And that actually sounded pretty good for once.

And Ross? What about him?

11

Training Journal of Emmy Wells

2/28	Wed.	3 Miles, Embarcadero, Pier 39.
3/2	Friday	3 Miles, Embarcadero, Pier 39.

Saturday, March 3, 6:45 am

We're doing another ten miler today. I'm dumping the Blowfish altogether and bringing my backpack (the Whale) instead. I hate that weight on my hips, so now I'm putting it on my back. And I'm loading it up with two bottles of Gatorade and a large water bottle. This time, I *will* stay hydrated.

Every time I walk with the team, it's a challenge. I have to stretch myself. But all week long I look forward to it. With the weight I've lost and with every new training walk, I get stronger, faster, and closer to walking up front with Kat and the others.

I want to do well today. I want to feel like I belong.

12

It was a small group and Emmy was glad. Everyone was relaxed; Tom and Michael joked as Marianne and Kat stretched with her, all of them laughing together. She felt good. And ready.

David retrieved his backpack and looked around for Juliette, but she didn't come running up late this time.

"Good morning!" he called out. "Today we're doing ten miles on the southern route. Who needs a map?" Emmy took one, but folded it up and put it away.* "We'll start with a walk along the Embarcadero to E4 and take our first break. Then it's Nob Hill by way of Clay Street. It's a long one, so pace yourselves. We'll go on to Lafayette Park for our second break. After that, we go straight west to the California Pacific Medical Center."

Emmy froze. *Oh, my God! No!* She couldn't breathe. A wave of nausea dizzied her and she fought for equilibrium. She shook her arms and listened closely to David's words.

"It's hallowed ground, ladies and gentlemen, one of the best breast

---

See Map on Page 323.

cancer treatment facilities in California, and they graciously allow us to take a break there. Please don't use the steps or railings to stretch and don't block the entrance. If a patient or visitor needs to use the restrooms, please let them go ahead of you."

He stopped and she couldn't take her eyes off his grim face. The medical center held a special meaning for him, too.

"Please," he asked, "be courteous. That's our final break, so I suggest you use it well. After that, we'll drop down along the Presidio, take the Pacific Street hill and head home."

Emmy didn't hear the safety rules. *California Pacific. Man, I don't want to go there.* Was there any way she could duck out? Maybe play sick? *No way.* She was in this thing now and all she could do was suck it up and go.

When they left, she started out next to Kat and walked in silence as they fought their way through tourists past Pier 39 and the ferry docks. She was going faster with Kat, so she settled into the silence and the speed, concentrating on her breathing and the rhythm of her steps. When David kicked the tempo up to four miles an hour, she was ready and kept her place beside Kat.

They reached E4 and Emmy immediately began to stretch. She knew her face was red. *Let everybody think it's the exertion.* Sweat dribbled on the concrete. David joined her and they stretched in silence. Why was the medical center so important to him? It must be the reason he was in the 3-Day. He must have lost someone to breast cancer—a sister maybe—or his mother. Or his *wife*. *Geez!*

They headed west through the Embarcadero Center, above the city streets. Open patios ran through the four buildings on three levels: Street, Lobby, and Promenade. Curving stairs led up and down between the levels, with shops along the way and elevated walkways connecting all four buildings. Stepping out into the sunshine, David led them up to the Promenade, then down the elevated walkway to E3, up the curved stairways again, then down the elevated walkway to E2, where Emmy worked. They walked steadily west—toward the medical center.

Emmy's stomach turned from sour to sick. It felt like the whole world swelled inside her and it was all hurt. She felt so full that she thought she might burst.

They shot past E1 and took the long stairway down over a burbling fountain to Street Level. David led them over to Clay Street, then stretched his way out in front, with Marianne and Tom right behind, Michael and Janet following, Kat and Emmy behind them, and Karen, Rhonda, Joy, Ellen, and ten other walkers.

As Clay Street turned into a hill, Emmy stayed with it every step of the way—until Chinatown. A red light stopped them at Powell and those ahead of them moved on up the hill. She paced back and forth, anxious to rejoin the others. Kat turned her head and stared pointedly at her.

When the light changed, Emmy shot across the street and attacked the hill. Her legs felt powerful, churning up the hill relentlessly. But it was a long hill. She had trained on shorter ones with steeper inclines, but Clay Street gradually went up, on and on and on. Forever.

The burn in her calves came hot and unexpected. David had said to pace yourself, but she hadn't listened. Falling back alongside Kat, she began to work the hill methodically. One foot in front of the other, until at last she heard applause and cheering. David and the others yelled and clapped as they topped the rise and stepped onto Taylor Street. Hands clapped her back. She heard Tom's laughter. Turning, she and Kat slapped a high five. She couldn't miss Kat's proud grin, but for Emmy it was just another damned hill done and gone.

Sweat poured off her. She stood silently, still expanded and full, staring out across the Bay at Alcatraz, and breathing deeply. Turning back to the group, she joined in clapping and cheering the walkers one by one as they made it to the top.

A black woman trudged at the end. She was way overweight. Sweat rolled off her arms in huge drops and her veins stood out against her skin, but she worked with a fierce determination. A moment later, she topped out, her face lit with joy. Emmy joined the others in clapping her on the back. She deserved it.

I can't believe what people give to this Walk. I just can't believe it.

"Great job, Bertina!" David called out.

Everyone took a moment to stretch and hydrate, then they turned and continued, downhill now, toward Van Ness, making a semi-circle from where they had started. When they reached the broad avenue, Bertina left them, heading back to Aquatic Park.

"She'll make it," David said, as if reading Emmy's thoughts. "I've never seen a woman so determined. I'll bet you anything she finishes every step of the 3-Day."

No sooner were they across the street than the next hill loomed before them. It was a short hill, but Emmy slowed down and fell back a bit, breathing evenly, working methodically, still with the front walkers. There was a final, deep push up concrete steps to the top. Her legs throbbed, but she topped out with no problem. Kat waited for her, a big smile on her face as she slapped Emmy's hand.

"Hell of a job!" she cried.

They walked past a tennis court and the break area was dead ahead. Emmy threw herself down on the grass and chugged Gatorade and water. A few minutes later, Michael slogged in, shimmering with sweat. He sat beside her and drank straight from a bottle of Gatorade, then pulled off his sweat band and squeezed it. About a pint of sweat ran out.

"Woo!" he cried. "That hill kicks some *serious* booty!"

The breeze was cool. Kat and Marianne joined them to stretch, but soon it was time to leave and they headed farther west. Every step felt heavier as she approached the medical center.

Memories pulsed through her: hours sitting on the little bench at the side of the door—walking home alone late at night—Dan, Amy's husband, fighting for breath—her mom's gross theatrics—the aching, the longing. She felt swollen with hurt, full up with it.

God, I don't wanna go back.

The approach was a long gentle incline, ever upward into the past. Over the last few blocks, laughter died away and conversations waned. It was as if they approached the gates of hell. Emmy walked by herself. Without momentum, she would have stopped altogether.

David and Marianne led them up the sidewalk to the entrance of California Pacific.

It was a three story building of light and dark pink stone on the north side of California Street. Two wide concrete steps with metal hand rails led up to double doors of clear glass.

Bile rose in Emmy's throat. She swallowed hard against it.

The door swung open and a girl stepped out, her face blotchy and tear-stained. David motioned for them to give the girl plenty of space. She turned aside, pacing up the side path to the little bench.

As the girl turned and sat, Emmy remembered Grace, sitting alone on the very same bench, weeping. It was where Emmy's dream had ended. It was where her memory was lost.

She took her place in line to wait for the bathroom, leaning back against the cool wall and closing her eyes. When her turn came up, she trudged in. She vividly remembered sitting here, during one of her visits, hugging herself, fighting against tears and winning. Dizziness returned. *I won't throw up. I won't cry.* She hugged herself tightly, gritted her teeth, and squeezed her eyes tightly closed.

I didn't cry then and I won't cry now.

Someone banged on the door.

"Emmy? Are you okay?" It was Kat.

"Yeah. I'll be out in a second."

She took a deep breath and opened the door. Kat was waiting, tense but quiet. They moved to the lawn and stretched. She caught David and Marianne glancing at her, but she focussed on stretching and working her legs hard until they felt good again.

If nothing else, she felt strong.

One more hill and then home.

They went back up California, then turned onto a side street. She was hardly aware of anything until David dropped back to walk beside her, then Marianne, walking on the other side. They were both quiet for a minute, then Marianne spoke:

"Brings back some bad memories."

"It's a tough place," David said.

They continued in silence and Emmy realized they were sharing memories of California Pacific. She was not alone. She was not alone any more. Her eyes welled up and it was all she could do to keep the tears inside.

Marianne reached over and rubbed her shoulder.

"It's always tough the first time back."

Emmy turned her head. It was hard to frame her question. "Did you... lose somebody?"

"No," Marianne answered, her eyes straight ahead. "It was my personal battleground. Twice walked in and twice walked out. It's hard not to think about it any time I get close."

"Twice? But you're so young."

Marianne laughed easily. "Thanks for the compliment. Actually, I'm thirty-two." *Geez!* She was the same age as Tina—and had it twice! "Breast cancer doesn't have an age restriction," she added. "It's a common misconception. I think all women should get mammograms, but then, I'm looking at it from a different place."

They were silent, then David glanced at Emmy.

"I lost somebody," he said. His voice was soft and there was no inflection, but she felt the pain. "I'm guessing you did, too."

It took a moment to clear her throat.

"Yes," she answered. "My aunt."

He leaned in to her, wrapping an arm around her shoulder. She slipped her arm around his waist and they walked together. Pushing up over the rise, they went steeply downhill to the alley where Pacific Street began.

David and Marianne moved forward to take the lead.

Emmy stood, staring up at it, and remembered Marianne's words. "You think you're home free and then there's this little monster that eats you alive." *Damn it! I've had it with little monsters that eat you alive.* Here was one that she could and would kill.

Stepping out, she ignored her aching legs and focussed on the task at hand. She used the techniques she knew by heart, but she was fueled by anger now.

Fuck this hill!

She walked faster and faster, passing Michael, Joy, and Ellen, then moving up past Tom and Kat. She pushed harder, working her way around Marianne until she walked side by side with David.

Through dripping sweat, he grinned at her.

They worked the hill together, like mismatched twins, David and Emmy against Goliath. Pushing on and on, they fought their way up. Her legs were powerful, her face set in grim determination. She pushed and pushed until suddenly they topped out.

David cried out, a primitive, inarticulate yell. Sweat poured from his doo-rag down through his glasses and Emmy felt her own sweat coating her body. He held up his hand and she slapped it, then lifted her face to the sky and whooped as loud as she could.

He turned to look down the hill and began clapping for Marianne and Kat, who grinned up at Emmy as they took the last few steps to the top. Laughing, she leaned against David.

The little monster was dead for another day.

13

Training Journal of Emmy Wells

4/13	Friday	3 Miles, Embarcadero, Pier 39.
4/14	Saturday	10 Mile Hill S. Route, Team Aquatic Park.
4/15	Sunday	15 Mile Hill, Team Aquatic Park.

Monday, April 16

Emmy couldn't work.

Knowing what day it was, Marcy had given her some computer graphics to play with, to keep her busy, but she just couldn't think. It was one year now, a full year to the day, and she couldn't think. Finally, she dragged herself to Marcy's door and peeked in.

"I gotta go," she said.

Marcy sighed and nodded. When Emmy had first applied at Markham Graphics, it was a real shock to find that both Jack

Markham, the owner, and Marcy, the lead graphic artist, already knew about her. Apparently, Amy had bragged her up enough that they hired her with barely a glance at her portfolio. Marcy knew. She understood.

"Go," she said. "You deserve a day off."

She shut down her computer, picked up her gym bag and the Whale, and headed for the bathroom. As she went by reception, Joanna looked up at her, but didn't say anything. After she had changed into her walking gear, she stopped back to drop off her gym bag and Tina was waiting.

"You're leaving?" she asked.

"Yeah. Need some time to myself," Emmy replied. She looked pointedly at Joanna as she handed over her gym bag. Joanna turned her eyes down and Emmy knew right away that she had called Tina.

"Are you okay?" Tina asked.

"Yeah, I'm fine," she lied. "I'm going for a walk. Okay?"

"Sure," Tina answered. "As long as you're sure."

The three women stared at each other in unspoken tension until finally Emmy smiled. *God, I love you guys,* she thought, *but a little mother-henning goes a long way.* She grinned.

"I'm sure." She hugged each of them warmly, then hefted the Whale to her back. She adjusted it to fit snugly. "I'll see you tomorrow, okay?"

Tina leaned forward and kissed her cheek.

"Be good."

"I will."

She turned to the elevator and rode down to Street Level. She quickly stretched and when she was ready, she turned her attention to the sidewalk.

Clay Street. David's route. It was good practice, especially since she had walked twenty-five miles over the weekend. Dodging pedestrians and bike messengers, she threaded her way up the hill toward Chinatown. She took small steps, stood erect, and regulated her breathing. Her legs were strong now and she felt the power.

It was now abundantly clear was that she couldn't keep stalling on her fundraising. She remembered how that guy from Pallotta had pounded away at fundraising, urging them to *double* or *triple* the minimum amount of nineteen hundred dollars. The whole purpose of the 3-Day was to raise money to fight breast cancer. It was now mid-April and she still hadn't asked one single person for a donation, including Ross or her family, all of whom would gladly contribute. Same with Tina and Joanna, who was a survivor herself.

It was time to formulate a plan.

And that meant she had to deal with Amy. Most of her donations would come from people who knew Amy—not just her old friends at Markham, like Jack and Marcy—but her personal friends, her associates, and her wealthy patrons. She would have to call Sandy, Amy's old personal assistant, to get a list of those patrons. She would have to pitch Mayor Willie Brown—he commissioned Amy's major public work. *Geez!* The mailing list would be enormous!

I really need a good letter.

She took the last few steps to the top of the hill, loosened the Whale and slung it off. She drank deeply from a Gatorade-spiked bottle and stretched again. There was mild pain, but it didn't bother her. She had trained the right way. She had eased into it and worked steadily to get strong, doing longer and harder walks until they were easy. She had learned from her teammates and grown.

She hefted the Whale to her shoulders and tightened it, then walked steadily down to Van Ness. Turning left, she walked to California Street. If she turned right, it would lead her past the one building she didn't want to see.

I'll take Pine Street today.

One year.

One year and counting since Amy died.

14

Training Journal of Emmy Wells

4/28	Saturday	13 Miles, Team Aquatic Park
4/29	Sunday	18 Miles, Team Aquatic Park
4/30	Monday	Rest.

Tuesday, May 1

After work, they picked up Chinese take-out and a six-pack of Tsingtao and headed to Ross's apartment. She had finally asked him to help her with fundraising and he was overjoyed. This was Ross in his element. He had asked her to take Wednesday off so she could ask for donations at Markham. She'd made appointments with the executives and planned to talk to the staff in between. Her stomach was so tied up in knots she didn't know how she'd eat.

She sat on the sofa with her box of Chinese veggies and steamed rice and Ross sat in his desk chair with sweet and sour shrimp, facing her across the coffee table.

"So what's your pitch?" he asked.

She hadn't thought about it, but it should be easy.

"I want to tell them all about the Walk and why I'm asking them for a donation and where the money goes." His shook his head so subtly that she barely caught the motion. "What?"

"You want my honest opinion, right?"

"Sure."

"That's like starting out two-thirds of the way through. You need to give it some context. Why are you walking, anyway? I mean, I know you're knocking yourself out with the training, but why? You need to start there."

Great. She had to start at the place she most want to avoid. He stopped eating and stared at her.

"Why?" he asked again.

Her fingers trembled. *I guess we'll have to talk about it sometime. Maybe sometime is now.* She cleared her throat. "I'm walking in memory of my aunt, Amelia Fleming."

His eyebrows shot up and his stare narrowed.

"*Amelia Fleming* was your aunt?"

"Yes."

"Wow!" he cried. "She died last year. Cancer, right?"

Emmy blew out a breath and met his eyes.

"Breast cancer."

"Holy shit! Emmy, God, I'm sorry."

Anger shot through her. She stood facing him.

"I don't need your pity, Ross. I don't need anybody's sympathy."

"Yes, you do. If you want them to donate, you need their sympathy. If they're not sympathetic to your cause, why should they donate?"

She stared at him. "They're already sympathetic. Everyone I'm asking for a donation knew Amy."

"Oh," he answered.

"Yes, oh!" Her voice was too loud, so she shut up and walked. It was one thing she was good at now. Unconsciously, her fingers tightened about the garnet heart at her neck.

He watched as she paced back and forth.

"So all you need is one simple statement." His voice was calm, soothing. "Something like, 'I'm walking in memory of my aunt, Amelia Fleming.' You just remind them. Give it context. The name conjures enough by itself, then go on and tell them what you're doing."

She stopped and stared at him, then quickly turned away. She didn't want to look in his eyes. He had learned something about her and he was walking on thin ice. She didn't like it at all.

"I'm sorry," she whispered.

"It's okay," he answered softly.

She had to turn this in a different direction.

"There's one thing I need your opinion on," she said. "At the end of the pitch, I want to ask them to double their donation. You think that would put them off?"

"No," he replied, nodding, "I think that's completely fair." She nodded and he nodded, then he looked up at her. "You wanted me to take a look at your letter?"

"Such as it is."

It took a moment to dig the three and a half inch floppy disk out of her purse. It was her "Amy Disk" and she had saved all of her drafts, photos, and email to this one place.

"There's a folder called '3-Day' with the drafts."

"Plural?"

"Yes. Open Number Seven."

While he looked it over, she took her cold veggies and rice into the kitchen, dumped them in a bowl, and stuck it in the microwave. It was really embarrassing to have such a bad letter after all this time, but Ross was the ad man. If he couldn't fix it, nobody could. He cleared his throat and she wandered back to peek over his shoulder as he worked. He had an earlier draft open and it looked like he'd been reading all of them. The microwave beeped.

Sitting down on the sofa, she ate as quickly as she could. She had learned many years ago that when you have a hole inside you, it's best to fill it as quickly as possible. That's how she got fat in the first place. She could trace it back to one day when she was thirteen years old. *Geez, five years ago.*

As she pushed in the last few bites, she noticed that Ross was working furiously. He had started a new file and was copying and pasting parts of her drafts, writing his own copy around them. She stood behind him, marveling at his speed.

"So some of it's useful?" she asked.

"Sure," he answered. "You had a good letter, just scattered over seven documents. The only thing that's missing is Amelia Fleming." He swiveled around to face her. "Are the letters going to people who knew her personally?"

"Some, but not all."

"More that knew her personally or didn't?"

The answer would determine how he phrased the Amy part of the letter. She wanted to lie, but couldn't.

"Mostly patrons, fans."

"Okay," he said, "let's tell them a little bit about her." He was quiet for a moment, then looked up at her. "I know this is hard for you, but try not to think about the aunt you loved. Think of her as a public figure, a well-known artist. Think of her in the abstract."

She nodded. He turned to the computer. Reaching over his shoulder, she picked up the box of cold sweet and sour shrimp. "Are you finished with this?"

"Yeah. Thanks." She gathered up the leftovers and took them into the kitchen, filling his fridge with stuff he might or might not eat in the coming days. It kept her busy. She didn't have to think about what he was doing.

It took a while, so she paced around, wondering what he could possibly write to "tell them about Amelia Fleming" when he never even met her.

I grew up with her. She taught me to draw.

As a child, Emmy had relied on Amy more than anyone she knew. With her overwrought mother constantly on the rampage, Aunt Amy offered calmness and continually radiated love. After her parents' divorce, Amy provided the only stability she had known. And during both of Amy's illnesses, they had spent many hours together, talking, laughing, their love deepening.

"I'm done," Ross called out. He swiveled to face her. "Let me read it to you." Walking back and forth, she noticed her hands were balled into fists, so she shook them out. "Maybe you'd better sit down," he added.

"Fine," she replied, walking around to sit on the sofa. She rested her hands on her knees. "Go ahead."

He turned to the computer and cleared his throat.

"'My aunt, Amelia Fleming, was first diagnosed with breast cancer in blank.' I need the date."

"October, 1994."

He typed it in, then swiveled around to face her.

"Ninety-four? That was seven years ago."

"Yes. You wanted her *first* diagnosis."

"She had it for seven years?"

"No! She had treatment. She was in remission for five years, then it came back. It's relentless that way, Ross. Don't you know anything about breast cancer?"

"No. I guess that makes me an ideal test dummy." He looked

perplexed for a moment, then turned back to the computer. "Maybe we should simplify this." He spoke as he typed. "How about, 'My aunt, San Francisco artist Amelia Fleming, died of breast cancer on blank.' What about that?"

Not bad. "It'll do."

"What's the blank?"

"April 16, 2000."

"'April 16, 2000.' Okay, that's enough." He paused as the date hit home. It had only been a little over one year. "New paragraph. 'This year, one out of every 13 women will face breast cancer.'" He continued reading from the new document and she let out her breath. He had organized her information beautifully and made a really good letter.

In that instant, she loved him.

"'That's why I'm walking sixty miles," he continued, "and that's why I'm asking you to donate to this cause. We simply must end breast cancer, so that women like Amelia Fleming can live long, fulfilling lives.' Period. What do you think?"

"It's great!"

In fact, it wasn't painful at all. It was abstract: it was Amy the famous, Amy the known. And there wasn't much of it, either—a little at the beginning, a little at the end.

She could deal with that.

"I saw a photo folder. You have pictures of her?"

"Yes, quite a few, actually."

"A photo at the top of the page would be really good. Mind if I take a look?"

"No, it's okay." Standing, she walked over behind him. "Use the one from her birthday party. It's my favorite."

He opened it up in his photo program, expertly resized it, and pasted it onto the top left of her letter. The opening blurb about Amy appeared to the right of it, but there wasn't enough text to make it look good. Too much white space. He moved back to the photo program, searching for a second photo to balance out the first.

Most of them weren't appropriate. There were many photos of Dan and Amy at their wedding, with Annie and Ben, their children, at the little lake on their property in the South Bay. There was a photo of them on their pontoon boat and many others.

But he opened the one picture she wished she didn't own. Her mom had taken it a few weeks before Amy's death. In her room at California Pacific, she lay asleep, her body wrecked and ravaged by the explosion of tumors that had metastasized into her lungs.

It was devastating.

She stood numbly as Ross resized it.

"Stop!" she cried. "You can't use that picture!"

The words were out before she could think. He froze, then turned in his chair to face her. He wrapped his arms around her waist, resting his head against her stomach.

"I'm sorry," he mumbled. She wrapped her arms around his head and buried her fingers in his hair where it fell around his collar. "I know it hurts," he said. Her eyes filled with tears, but she closed them tightly. *I will not cry.* "This *will* raise more money," he said, looking up at her. "I'm *with* you. We need to end breast cancer. Abstract. Think of it in the abstract."

She swallowed and nodded.

Disentangling himself, he swiveled around and moved the photo into place on the opposite side of the letter. The text nestled neatly above the two pictures, but he played with it a moment longer so it read: "On April 16, 2000, my aunt, San Francisco sculptor Amelia Fleming, died of breast cancer."

"Geez!" she said. The word was little more than a breath. She was dying inside, but she knew he was right. "It may alienate some people," she protested weakly. "It's like hitting them over the head with a giant hammer!"

"But it works."

"Yes," she answered. "Save it. Print out fifty copies for me to take along tomorrow."

15

Training Journal of Emmy Wells

5/1 Tues. 3 Miles, Embarcadero, Pier 39.

Wednesday, May 2, 8:45 am

The day is off to a good start. I've already talked to three people and collected forty-five dollars. I started with Paul, partly because he's sympathetic and partly because we're pretty relaxed together, having worked in the same cubicle for eight months. I flubbed a few things, but it was good to get my jitters out of the way early. My target with Paul was ten dollars and he came through with twenty, so that was great.

Even so, I'm completely wracked about seeing Jack Markham. He is the Owner. President. CEO. Amy's friend. My appointment is for 9, so I only have 15 minutes of terror yet to go.

16

She stood in front of Tina's desk, both of them watching the phone, waiting for the line to clear.

In her hands, she held a large, brown envelope with Jack's letter and five donation forms. She had already given two forms to Tina, one for the company match that Jack had all but promised (nine-hundred and fifty dollars, half the total) and one for his personal donation. Tina would fill them out for him.

When the extension light winked off, she nodded to Emmy, then buzzed him on the intercom.

"Yes?" he asked through the speaker.

"Emmy Wells is here to see you."

There was a brief silence, then he cleared his throat.

"Send her right in."

As she approached the door, he opened it for her. His smile was sad as he ushered her over to his casual area. She sat on the sofa and he sat across from her.

"Before we talk about money," he said, "I just want to say I totally support what you're doing. Amy and I were friends for over twenty years, all the way back to Stanford. She was a very special person and it was really hard to lose her."

Right to the point. It flustered her.

"Thanks," she mumbled, "I appreciate it."

"It was tough," he said, "very tough." Her throat swelled up. *Geez.* She didn't want to talk about Amy. "I remember when you interviewed here," he continued, "you told me she taught you how to draw with your crayons." He smiled sadly. Emmy steeled herself. She didn't want to think about that. *I've got to push on.* Somehow, she had to make the conversation about the 3-Day.

"Unfortunately, this isn't just about Amy," she said, lifting her voice. "Last year, in the United States, over fifty thousand women died from breast cancer—and hundreds of thousands had mastectomies."

It was jerky, but at least she got it out.

"I didn't realize!" He sounded genuinely alarmed. Then it hit her: Julia! She had met his wife at the Christmas party...

Okay, let's go.

"Has Julia—" she couldn't finish the question.

His eyes grew round. "No, thank God. No!" he answered. His voice faltered and he looked everywhere but at Emmy.

She panicked. *God, don't let me blow this!*

"I'm glad," she said. "Yes. Thank God."

"Yes." Finally, he looked at her again. "I'm astounded at how brave women are. Especially Amy."

She moved forward on the sofa. They were totally off script and she had to get him away from Amy so she blurted it out:

"I'm walking in the Breast Cancer 3-Day."

He nodded. It was all the encouragement she needed.

"There's about twenty-five hundred of us and we'll be walking sixty miles from San Jose to San Francisco to raise money for breast cancer research and outreach programs."

"Yes," he replied. His voice was full of relief. He was just as glad as she that they had moved on. "Tina's told me all about it. I'm proud of you. The whole company's behind you. We're matching half of your required amount, nine-hundred and fifty dollars."

"Thanks, Jack, I really, really appreciate it."

"It's the least we can do," he replied. "You represent the firm. You'll be walking for all of us, you know."

He shifted his weight, as if he was about to stand and end the interview, but she didn't move. She looked into his eyes and held him there for a long moment, then pulled her letter from the brown envelope.

"I'm very thankful for the company donation, but I'm asking you to make a personal donation, too. I'd really appreciate it if you'd read this letter asking for your financial support."

She handed him the letter. When he saw the two pictures of Amy side by side, she heard him suck in a breath. He seemed genuinely moved, seeing his dear friend so seriously ill. He read Emmy's plea for a donation and, for a moment, she didn't see the businessman—she saw a human being—someone who had lost a close friend. He moistened his mouth and cleared his throat.

"Of course, I'll make a personal donation."

Standing, he walked briskly to a bulletin board and tacked the letter up for his visitors to see. He turned to his desk, opened his briefcase, and removed a checkbook. He sat. Lifting an expensive pen, he held it poised over a check. It was time for Emmy to play her trump card. Standing, she walked to his desk.

"Before you write the check," she said, "I want you to know how much this means to me. Whatever amount you were thinking of donating, I want you to consider doubling it." He looked up at her. "I'm serious," she continued. She sat down, holding his eyes. "It's probably too much to ask, but I've got to do everything I can to find a cure. As I said, it isn't just about Amy. It's about Julia, too. And Tina and Joanna.

Who knows, maybe even me some time." *Me?* She shivered and her voice wavered. "Breast cancer can kill anyone."

He cleared his throat and stared at the checkbook.

"Who's it payable to?"

"Avon Breast Cancer 3-Day. And Jack—regardless of the amount—thanks."

He smiled and wrote the check. Looking down at the floor, she breathed out. She'd done it. She couldn't see what he was writing, but he executed it with a certain flair. He tore out the check and walked around his desk. She stood facing him.

"For what it's worth," he said in a quiet voice, "I *did* double the amount. And it's from the heart." He handed her the check.

Two hundred dollars!

"Thanks!"

He put his hand on her shoulder and walked her to the door. "I appreciate what you're doing," he said. "Thank *you*."

"Oh, before I go—" she pulled out the remaining forms. "Would you mind giving these to some of your friends?"

He laughed, a single short bark, and took them.

"I'll give them to Julia—I'm sure she'll encourage her friends to donate. Good luck with your walking."

The door closed behind her and she hustled over to Tina's desk. Both forms were already filled in, except for the amount listed on Jack's personal donation. Emmy held up the check and Tina grinned as she filled it in.

"We still on for lunch?" she asked.

"You bet. Don't forget your checkbook."

It was a good beginning, but it was just a beginning. *Almost twelve hundred dollars. Only seven hundred left to reach the minimum.* She went from office to office and desk to desk. She varied her pitch from person to person and kept it fresh. For those she didn't know well, she stressed the statistics and the difficulty of walking sixty miles. Sometimes she talked about the training, but sometimes, as with Jack, she left it out. But she asked for double the donation from everyone. It was hard to tell if it worked because she didn't know what people were planning to give, but she collected a donation from everyone—and met or exceeded her target amount.

The VP was traveling, but his Assistant pledged a hundred dollars on his behalf and added twenty of her own. The Comptroller reluctantly donated another hundred. Everyone else gave between ten and fifty.

By noon, She had collected sixteen hundred and thirty-five dollars and still had at least half the company to go, including all of the project managers and most of the support staff. Of course, she would get smaller donations from them, but that was okay. She was getting very close to her goal.

Joanna and Tina met her at reception and they went to a trendy restaurant near the Bank of America Building. Emmy had decided not to use a letter with either of them. It wouldn't be fair to show them the picture of Amy, especially at lunch. In fact, she wondered if she should ask them to donate at all, but she knew she had to. And they were expecting it.

Tina ordered her usual martini, while Joanna sipped iced tea. Emmy looked across the table at Tina.

"Can I ask a personal question?"

Tina smiled back. "Anything you want."

"Have you ever had a lump in your breast?"

She laughed. "Breasts, honey—and no, my breasts are good." As if to emphasize her point, she adjusted her bra and grinned. Emmy glanced over at Joanna. The older woman's lips crinkled at the corners as she stared at Tina.

"Ever had a mammogram?" she asked.

"No!" Tina cried. "But I've heard stories. Sounds awful. My doctor says I shouldn't need them for another ten or twenty years. Thank goodness!"

Pursing her lips, Emmy stared down at the table top.

"What?"

"I want you to be careful," she said. "I met this woman on one of my training walks. Marianne. She's only thirty-two—same as you—but she's had breast cancer twice." She looked into Tina's eyes to see if her message was getting across. It was: the flippant smile had disappeared and Tina's eyes were wide open. "I know," Emmy continued, "most women your age don't get it, but I'm just saying... be careful. Learn how to do a self-exam. Make sure you stay safe."

It may have put a damper on lunch, but it was good to see Tina taking it seriously. Before they left the restaurant, Tina wrote a check for fifty dollars and Joanna contributed another fifty, much more than Emmy had expected.

From their many conversations working together, Marcy already knew what she was doing and why, so Emmy decided to keep her approach simple. She knocked on the door and Marcy waved her in.

"My turn for the grist mill?"

"What?" Emmy sat in the chair in front of her desk.

"Word has it your pitch is kind of gruesome."

Wow. She hadn't considered that people would talk about it, but she should have expected it. Small company, big gossip.

"Sorry," she said. "I didn't mean for it to come off so grim. I don't want to make people feel bad."

"It's okay," Marcy replied. "It can't be easy for you—and I certainly understand why you're doing it."

"Well, I'm not gonna give you a pitch. You know I'm asking for a donation. You know why. But I *would* appreciate it if you read my letter."

"Okay."

She pulled it from her envelope and passed it over, along with a donation form. Marcy slipped on her reading glasses and took a long look at the letter. She studied the pictures carefully and mumbled, "Geez." When she was finished, she leaned back in her chair and closed her eyes. She had been very close to Amy, too.

"Can I use my credit card?" she asked.

"Sure," Emmy answered. "There's a space at the bottom of the form where you can fill everything in. You can also mail it in, if you want, or give it to me later."

"Thanks. You want twice what I was going to give?"

Emmy nodded. "We need to raise as much money as we can. I

don't have to tell you how important it is." They stared at each other across the desk. Emmy smiled. "I'll beg if I have to."

Marcy laughed. "You don't have to beg. I'll donate a hundred dollars." Lifting the donation form, she looked at the credit card section. "I'll get this back in an hour."

"Thanks! I really appreciate it."

Emmy stood up to leave, but Marcy stopped her.

"Emmy?"

"Yes?"

"Just between two women in the ad business, you might want to watch the hard sell." She waved the letter. "It works with some people, but this is pretty grim. Be careful."

"Thanks, Marcy. I will."

After speaking to everyone in what they called the "work section," the artists, designers and project managers, she was finished for the day. It was a little after four o'clock. At her desk, she counted up the donations:

Two thousand, three hundred and fifteen dollars.

She had passed her minimum in less than eight hours! All that stress and tension for a mere eight hours of work! Grinning, she stuffed all of her donations in the brown envelope and packed up the Whale.

Grabbing her gym bag, she headed to the restroom to change into her walking clothes. Down at Street Level, she quickly stretched, adjusted the Whale on her back, then headed for the 3-Day office on Market Street. A year ago, she never would have thought of walking this distance, but as she pushed up the sidewalk, dodging in and around people, she walked right by three BART stations, yet her Fast Pass remained firmly in her wallet.

After dropping off her donations, she headed toward Pine Street and the new route home from work.

Try as she may, Emmy just couldn't suppress the smile that had taken over her face. *Look at what I did!* She had started out in January over-weight, sluggish, unmotivated, and—*let's face it*—depressed, but since then—since she'd started training—she'd lost sixteen pounds, she'd grown stronger and she'd grown to love walking. Now she was dedicated to something.

Last Sunday, I walked eighteen miles.

Eighteen miles! Unbelievable. Unthinkable.

She grinned.

And now, she'd met the minimum fundraising requirement on her very first day! She knew she could bring in a lot more. Now that she'd met the minimum, her next goal was to *double* it. Thirty-eight hundred dollars. To do that, she would have to raise fifteen hundred dollars from her friends, her acquaintances in the business world, artists and dealers that worked with Amy, her classmates, her teachers, her high school friends, her neighbors, her mother's neighbors, Mayor Willie Brown, the governor—whoever she could reach!

It was impossible to contain her happiness.

Maybe it was time to talk to Barb about terminating her therapy. It was time to move on. She wasn't a child any more.

Starting up the Pine Street hill, she shortened her stride and breathed in a steady rhythm. In through the nose, out through the mouth, one foot in front of the other, until she topped out. Slinging the Whale off her back, she drank from her Gatorade-spiked water.

This coming Sunday, she would walk twenty miles and she felt ready. David had escalated their base walks from seven to ten to thirteen miles. She was a member of a great team and the tie that bound David and the others now encircled her, too.

Hefting the Whale to her back, she turned on her heel and set off down the street.

At the end of June, they would do a complete simulation, then, at the end of July, the Big Kahuna. Sixty miles in three days. Twenty-five hundred women and men dedicated to the task of erasing breast cancer from the face of the earth.

A middle aged woman, pushing a shopping cart, sourly regarded her, as if perplexed by Emmy's trek. It reminded her of the day she saw David Cook walking alone up Van Ness Avenue. And here she was, marching alone up Pine. And now she knew what drove him. Like her, he had lost someone he loved deeply. And maybe that someone had been the love of his life.

He had always seemed the most alone of everyone in the group, but they shared something now. *From now on,* she decided, *I'll be his friend, not just another walker for him to look after, but a real friend.*

Turning, she strode west down Pine Street.

She walked alone.

She walked fast.

And she walked with a definite sense of purpose.

17

Training Journal of Emmy Wells

5/5	Saturday	13 Miles Team Aquatic Park.
5/6	Sunday	20 Miles Team Aquatic Park.

Tuesday, May 8

"So, what do you think?" Emmy asked. "Everything's going great. I feel really good. I think we should just finish this up and I can get on with my life and you'll have room for somebody who really needs you."

Barb raised her eyebrows and gave a little shake of her head. It was unconscious. Emmy had seen her do it before when she was absorbing information she wasn't prepared to process. Her short brown hair floated a centimeter left, then back again.

"That's wonderful!" she said. "It sounds like your life couldn't be better." Something about the way she said it made Emmy think she didn't really believe it. "Let's see. Of course, your walking is going great. I can't believe you walked thirty-three miles in one weekend!"

Emmy winced as she heard the words spoken aloud. *Geez, it sounds like a lot, but I earned it. Every damn mile.* The pain never went away.

"You've lost sixteen pounds. You've raised—what did you say? Almost three thousand dollars?" Emmy nodded. Barb smiled. "I think this is working out very well. You seem to be happy with your boyfriend, your classes, your job."

She raised her eyebrows again, as if to ask if she had left anything out. Emmy just smiled back at her.

"Yeah, it's great."

"What about your father?"

"I'm okay with him. Grace is okay with him. Of course, Dean isn't. Not Mom. Maybe you should start seeing *Mom*."

Barb smiled. "That's between us." She winked at Emmy. "When was the last time you *saw* your father?"

"Um... January."

"I remember. He took you out for dinner and gave you *money* for your birthday."

"You say that like it's a bad thing. Come on. He lives in Livermore for goodness sake. It's half-way across the state. He's got his own family now. Besides, he already gave me the best gift on my twelfth birthday."

Barb glanced at the garnet heart. It was Emmy's birth stone. She'd worn it every day since her dad gave it to her. Unconsciously, she now took it between her fingers.

Barb stared at her until she had to look away.

"Has he called? Have you called him?"

"No. I'm fine with that. He sends a check every month with a little note. Love you. Miss you. That kind of thing."

"But he never apologized. You've never forgiven him."

"He's not the one I need to forgive, remember?"

"You've already forgiven Dean. Or so you said. Unless you're thinking about your mother."

Her words ignited something in Emmy and the anger came fast and hard. She had felt so good when she'd sat down. Barb just had a way of messing everything up. She dug into things that didn't really matter. *Some therapist!*

"Why would I have to forgive Mom?"

Barb shrugged. "When you talk about her, you always sound angry. You've called her weak, stupid, hysterical, Irish, a crybaby... completely out of control." She paused to think. "Witchy. I forgot witchy."

A lump formed in Emmy's throat. She opened her mouth, but only whispered, "She's not Amy."

Barb sat quietly, tipping her pen against her pursed lips, then looked steadily into Emmy's eyes.

"I think losing Amelia was *like* losing your mother."

Emmy swallowed the lump and shook her head. She would *not* let the conversation go there. When she spoke, it was hard to control her anger.

"What does it matter? She's gone. I'm doing this Walk for her. And it's *not* all rosy. I walk with women who've had breast cancer over and over, people who've lost their loved ones. Yes, it's good and I have fun, but I've got to live with this shit all the time." She stopped. Everything she had that was good was gone. *Damn!*

"You say you're walking for your aunt Amelia," Barb said slowly, "but you don't want to talk about her. I don't think you've faced her death yet—in a *concrete* way." She sat back in her chair, regarding Emmy with steely eyes. "I have an assignment for you."

Emmy closed her eyes and swallowed hard. For the first time all day, she felt sick.

"I've done some research on these walks. It's common for people to create a *memorial* shirt to wear and they get all of their loved ones to sign it. I want you to create a shirt in memory of Amelia Fleming. I want you to get it signed and I want you to wear it one of the three days."

Emmy's stomach turned over.

Will I ever put this behind me?

18

Training Journal of Emmy Wells

5/10	Thursday	3 Miles, Embarcadero, Pier 39.
5/11	Friday	3 Miles, Embarcadero, Pier 39.

Friday, May 11, 4:50 pm

Well, I did it. I bought a pink, long-sleeved tee shirt, simple, unadorned. My memorial shirt. I took it to a print shop, with a photo—the picture from Amy's birthday party—for the back. It's stunning. I selected a minimum of words for the front, to be printed in black ink:

AMELIA FLEMING

October 20, 1959—April 16, 2000

I'll wear the shirt on Day Two. I'll be so focussed on Hell Hill that it shouldn't bother me.

Anyway, the order is in. Abstract. I get it.

19

Training Journal of Emmy Wells

5/12 Saturday 13 Miles Team Aquatic Park.

Sunday, May 13

In the blackness of her sleep, she heard the slap of her shoes as she walked along a sidewalk. Her feet, under the blankets, twitched with the motion.

Warmth spread through her body and a spike of elation jolted her dream. Sweat rolled down her cheeks and she felt simply lost in the joy of walking. Then she saw the doors of California Pacific and the path at the side of the building. Grace sat, tears marking her face.

Emmy felt an intense pain in her stomach, as if all the sludge in the world had massed there and started growing worms. She grabbed her belly. The pain turned to panic.

She took another step as the fear overwhelmed her. It was about to drag her under and she knew a blackout was imminent. Bracing herself, she took another step. Then another, on up the steps toward the entrance.

Pain roared through her. She stood before the door, the reflection a portrait of her younger self. She reached out to push the door and felt so terrified that all of her muscles tightened and then violently exploded.

Her leg kicked out in one great spasm and hit something hard.

"Ow! God damn it!"

Ross twisted in the darkness. Coated in sweat, Emmy sat up, gasping for air. Ross jumped from the bed and banged against something.

"Jesus Christ!"

The lamp clicked on. Rubbing his leg, Ross squinted at her in the dim light.

"Damn!"

Her heart pounded as she realized she'd recovered part of her lost memory. If she hadn't awakened, she might have opened the doors. But now she didn't want to recover the memory. She didn't want to know what would happen when she opened the doors.

Suddenly, the alarm clock beeped. Reaching down to slap it off,

Ross peered at the digital readout.

"Four-fifteen! Jesus! Emmy? You okay?"

She blew out a breath. "Yeah. It was just a dream."

Rising from the bed, she hobbled into the bathroom. She tried to be quick because he would be waiting, like always. He'd been so crabby lately. Of course, he hated getting up early to give her a ride, but lately he'd been giving her crap about how much time she gave to the 3-Day, like she had a choice. Training and fundraising were where she lived right now. In a few months it would all be over and they could get back to normal.

If they *could* get back to normal. If there *was* a normal.

On the other hand, she had to walk. If there was one thing she absolutely had to do, it was walk. It was true that she'd been consumed with putting together mailing lists and printing donation letters, but she had to get it done. She even finished early last night so they could watch some stupid zombie movie and that was a total disaster.

She left the bathroom and Ross rushed in right behind her. It pissed her off. Everything pissed her off. Either *she* was mad or *he* was mad and it just plain sucked. She quickly dressed, then, sitting on the bed, she put on a pair of her favorite old ankle socks, laced up her shoes, and slipped on her thermal pants.

It was a big day and she had to be at her best. Twenty-three miles—for the first time—almost the same distance as Day One. The twenty-miler the previous Sunday had killed her, but she knew it would help on this one. Muscle memory.

God, I hope I'm ready.

She threaded her hair through the hole of her baseball cap. Snatching up the Whale, she hustled into the kitchen and loaded in two large bottles of Gatorade and two waters from the fridge. She turned to the kitchen table and looked in the fruit basket. Her banana was missing! She'd saved one banana for the walk. Glancing around the room, she noticed the peel in the trash. *Ross ate it!*

Growling, she took an apple instead. *God damn it!* Maybe they needed some time apart. It might sober him up—and she could do without the aggravation. *I'm really glad I didn't move in with him.*

The bathroom door opened and she went back to take a final pee. *Get as much out as possible.* They met at the door and she slipped on her windbreaker. He picked up the box of letters she had finished right before the zombie movie.

"I'll drop these off at the post office," he said, "as soon as the rest of the world is awake."

He locked the door and they started down the hall.

"*Somebody* ate my banana."

"*Your* banana?" He looked at her in surprise. "Really. I'm pretty sure I bought the bananas."

"You know I like to take one with me on walks. There was only one left."

"Sorry," he replied, sounding anything but. "I must have been so dazed at getting kicked in the middle of the night that I didn't even notice."

They waited for the elevator in silence. "Sorry about that," she said after a bit. "I had a shitty dream. Remind me to never watch another zombie movie. Or eat buttered popcorn."

"Got it," he answered. "I'll add 'em to the list."

She glanced at him. No one did cynical better. They were silent going down to the car and quiet through the short drive. *This is so messed up,* she thought. *Maybe we should have a talk this afternoon after the Training Walk.*

When they arrived at Aquatic Park, she turned to him.

"See you around noon?"

"I'll be here," he answered.

Slipping out of the car, she started toward the bleachers. Two words sarcastically floated up behind her.

"You're welcome."

Stopping, she gritted her teeth and turned to thank him, but it was too late. He threw the Scoupe into gear, roared around the turnaround and raced away. *Damn it! How did this get started? Things shouldn't be this way.* They cared about each other. Why should he be hurtful? They used to have a really good thing and now she just felt awful.

Turning on her heel, she faced the early morning darkness; the lights on the Maritime Museum provided only dim illumination. Slowly, she picked her way to the bleachers.

"Hey, guys," she called out as she skipped up the steps.

"Morning, Emmy," David said, echoed by others.

"Good luck finding the sign-in sheet," Tom remarked.

She found it, but had to tilt it to the light to sign in. Her eyes were slowly adjusting to the darkness. She found Kat and they stretched together.

"You ready for this?" Kat asked.

"As ready as I'll ever be."

"Wait till we do the simulation," Marianne said. "Then you'll be ready."

"Has David scheduled it yet?"

"Last two days of June and first of July. Friday, Saturday and

Sunday. We're starting at eight, so we won't be back till mid-afternoon. You'll get a ticket if you park in the lot."

"Same routes as last year?" Kat asked.

"Yep. Twenty-three miles on Friday, sixteen on Saturday and twenty on Sunday. Then, we cut distance for three weeks."

"Why's that?" Emmy asked.

"Recuperation. The sim will kick your ass."

As they talked, the bleachers filled up with walkers. *Just what we need today—a full load.* It was just one more thing. Too many things. She was so tired. Everything was messed up. Even walking was so damn painful. And losing weight. She hated being hungry all the time, craving ice cream and fried chicken and buttered popcorn. It was driving her crazy.

"I don't care!" A girl's voice, back at the entrance.

"Here we go." Marianne stepped briskly toward the sound, with Tom right behind her. Angling her body to get a look at what was going on, Emmy listened closely.

"I'm sorry, Lauren, you can't do it," David said.

The sky was milky in the east and she could see a little better. He was talking to a bald girl who looked like she was about fourteen.

"I'm a registered walker," Lauren answered in a strong voice. "No one can stop me from training."

"It's a twenty-three miler," Marianne replied. "You know what those are like."

There were two other girls, one on each side of Lauren.

"We'll help," the blond one said.

"That's what we're here for," the other one added.

"I've gone as far as sixteen miles already," Lauren said. "I'm fit. I can make it."

Kat sighed.

"What's that all about?" Emmy asked.

"Lauren," Kat answered. "She walked with us last year, but she's just finishing her third round of chemo—in the last four years. David doesn't want her to walk at all."

Emmy stared at her. *How could that little girl even consider walking?*

"She's had breast cancer three times?"

"It runs in the family. She's lost her mother and grandmother. Hell, Lauren's already had two mastectomies." She stood and peered at the group by the entrance. "She's a tough kid, I'll give her that. She won't give up."

"She doesn't look old enough to qualify."

"Yeah, she looks young, but she's twenty-two."

"Okay," David said, "but if you can't finish, I'll count on your friends to get you back here." All three of the girls nodded. He picked up the clipboard and walked it back to them. They signed in and passed it back to him. Other walkers, who had arrived late, waited down on the sidewalk.

"Alright, everybody!" he called out as he turned to the group. "I'm closing the walk. We have thirty-six walkers and that's all we can take today. If you got here late, stick around for a minute. As you all know, we're doing twenty three miles today. The time limit in the parking lot expires at noon, so that's our goal to get back here. If you do the math and factor in six ten minute breaks, we're looking at averaging four miles an hour. Every time we get a long, flat stretch, we'll be walking as fast as we can to make up for the time we lose on hills. *Twenty-three miles* with *four big hills* at *four miles an hour*. If anybody can't pull that load, now is the time to bow out.

"Please come up and scratch your name off the list."

Hell, that scares me*—and I'm more or less used to it.*

Six people came forward to scratch, so he motioned to those waiting on the sidewalk and six more people stepped up to replace them, including Juliette, who was late, as usual.

David turned back to face his walkers, grinning. "The rest of you are nuts!" Nervous laughter swept across the bleachers. "Who needs a map?"

Since she hadn't done twenty-three miles before, Emmy took one.*

At the end of the safety lecture, David stopped and looked everyone over. "Listen close for a minute. This is gonna be a tough walk. If anybody gets dizzy or dehydrated, we need to know about it immediately. Pay attention to those around you."

He glanced at Emmy.

"Somebody may not realize they need help. Be a lifeline for each other. And always remember the safety motto." Emmy joined her voice with the others in speaking the slogan aloud: "Stay Alert, Stay Alive."

At the stroke of five, they moved out toward Pier 39. Kat and Emmy took their place behind Marianne and Janet. The warm-up period was short. Since they didn't have to dodge street vendors, David upped the pace very early. There was no chatter as they hustled along. The only sound was air sucked in and blown out. Within a half mile, the regulars outdistanced the newcomers.

---

* See Map on Page 355.

Arriving at E4, coated in sweat and gasping for air, there was the usual rush for the bathrooms. Emmy could wait this time, so she started to stretch. As she bent down, Bertina trotted up the stairs, looking considerably thinner and breathing evenly. As David had predicted, she'd turned into a hell of walker and it really made Emmy feel good.

Lauren and her two friends trudged up the stairs just minutes later. They were doing well. Although Lauren was thin, her muscles were well toned. *How on earth can she train while doing chemo?* As Lauren pulled off the bandana that she wore around her bald head, they made eye contact. She smiled, then squeezed out the sweat. Emmy nodded to her and received a nod in return.

She stored her thermal pants and windbreaker in the Whale and she was ready to go. David marched them through the Embarcadero Center and across the skyways all the way to Clay Street and it was almost a relief to face the hill.

Slowing down, they paced themselves. Bertina was right behind Emmy topping the hill and they slapped a high-five. As soon as the whole team was assembled, David turned to Marianne.

"Time to split up?"

"I'd say so," she answered. "I'll take the slow group first." They each took out a cell phone and turned them on. "I'll call you when we hit Lafayette Park."

"Okay," David replied. "See you at California Pacific."

Without further discussion, he turned and headed down the street. Marianne stayed behind, encouraging the slower walkers behind them up the hill.

They moved fast again all the way down to Van Ness, then worked their way briskly up the hill to Lafayette Park. Leaning against a bench, Emmy stretched her calves as the first rays of sunshine broke across the treetops. She was so tired already. Not enough sleep. Scary dreams. It added up.

Lauren stretched out on the grass to work her hammies and Emmy watched her. It was crazy what that girl had to face—it made her own little problems seem petty. Somehow, in the haze of training and fundraising, she had forgotten what was important. Lauren's skin was pale. She was tired, too, but her eyes were fierce with life.

Pushing herself up from the bench, Emmy walked over and offered her hand. "Emmy," she said.

"Lauren." They clasped hands and Lauren pushed herself up as Emmy pulled. "Nice to meet you."

"I admire what you're doing," Emmy said.

"Thanks," Lauren replied, smiling. "I appreciate what you're doing, too. We're all in it together."

As she let go of Lauren's hand, she looked into her eyes. "Be careful," she whispered. "David knows what he's talking about."

Lauren laughed easily. "Believe me," she answered, "I know. I'll be careful. Besides, I've got my guardian angels." Her friends stepped up beside her. This is Alex," she said, hooking her thumb at the blond. "And Darla."

"Let's get moving," David called out.

Juliette fell in beside Emmy and they pushed each other to keep pace behind Kat and Tom. She couldn't stop thinking about Lauren. Her mother. Grandmother. Life felt so precious, every breath so precious. *And somehow I screwed it all up!* But she should be able to fix it. She had to make things right with Ross. She'd never seen him like he was that morning, peeling out of the parking lot. Why was he driving her anyway? If he let her use the Scoupe, she could drive and he could sleep in. That would solve one problem.

It was also time to put fundraising aside, except for a bake sale she had planned with her mother and Grace, then just zero in on training. Get things back to normal with Ross.

That was a plan. It was a good plan. Very doable.

Looking up, she saw California Pacific down the block. They were already half-way across the City, almost a third of the way through this walk. She could do it. Hell, she'd done twenty miles already. *Just focus on the walk.* She got out of the bathroom just as Lauren and her guardian angels arrived. They were falling further behind.

David closed his phone and looked at Emmy.

"Marianne says they're about ten minutes behind."

Her legs were stiff, so she joined Kat on the grass to do some serious stretching. Across the lawn, Tom erupted in laughter. She had never seen anyone who laughed so much.

"Why's he always so happy?" she asked.

Kat chuckled. "That's one of his jokes," she replied. "And in his case, it's true. 'Why is that man always so happy?' Answer? 'He's a gynecologist!'"

"For real?"

"For real! And do yourself a favor, don't get him started on gynecologist jokes. He can go on for hours."

When Emmy looked up, Marianne approached with the second group and switched places with Janet. David gave her a few minutes to stretch and hydrate, then they moved out again, continuing west at high speed, up through a gate into the Presidio.

They passed the old Marine hospital, site of her earlier dehydration meltdown, made a complete loop around the back of the golf course in a circle that brought them to Mountain Lake.

As Emmy sat stretching, Lauren and her two friends slowly walked into the break area. The girl was very pale and worn. She was done. Eleven miles and three hills—two of them extremely long—had been too much. The three girls stretched for while, then turned and began their difficult trek back to Aquatic Park. Emmy looked at David, who shrugged as he shouldered his backpack.

"Lots more miles to go," he said.

Emerging from the Presidio, they headed west. Walking up a long gentle incline, the pace slowed a little and Tom fell back to walk beside her. They had never talked much, but the fact that he was a gynecologist made her curious.

"So," she said, "what brings you to the 3-Day?"

He glanced at her sideways, but he wasn't smiling. Through his horn-rimmed glasses, she saw the eyes of a serious and thoughtful man.

"I'm walking for a former patient of mine," he answered, "a family friend. Jessica Timmons. I delivered her two baby girls." He was silent for a minute as he looked at the sidewalk in front of him. "She died two years ago." He shook his head. "Now, those girls are motherless. It's not fair."

They turned toward Point Lobos.

"What about you?" he asked. "How come you're walking?"

Well, there it was again.

When will I ever learn to keep my big mouth shut?

"My aunt. She died last year."

"Sorry," he said, turning his head to look into her eyes. "We really need to find a cure, huh?" She smiled at him and they picked up their speed to catch up with the others.

Finally, they crested the hump of the hill and she saw the Pacific Ocean spreading forever behind the Cliff House. It was so beautiful she wanted to cry. She didn't even see this view on the twenty mile walk. She'd just tried to survive it.

They walked down the long, curving sidewalk toward the ocean. Her hips and back hurt badly, but her feet were so swollen that her shoes felt deadly tight. She considered changing socks and powdering her feet, but she was so tired. All she wanted was rest.

Slipping between the hot dog stand and the restaurant, she and Kat hurried down the concrete steps to the bathrooms, then braced themselves against the sea wall. They looked out on the ocean as they stretched. Every now and then, a large wave pounded against the rocks below and a little spray blew over them.

A wave of sadness passed over her again. There was a time when she visited Cliff House to sketch and she missed that very much. With everything going on—school, work, walking, fundraising, Ross, therapy—she hadn't been here in months.

It was time to start getting *everything* back in order.

They spent the whole break at the sea wall, then walked up the stairs to join the others. David's cell rang. Janet's group was so far behind that they had to turn around and go back to avoid parking tickets. When he got off the phone, he looked up at them.

"Better get moving."

They followed the sidewalk down along Ocean Beach and then across Great Highway into Golden Gate Park. Walking along in the cool shade of the trees, Emmy felt a burning on the ball of her right foot. The pain was slight, so she thought she could fix it. Stopping, she pulled up her socks, retied her laces, and set out again, but it hurt worse. Each step became so painful that she had to limp.

She slowed down and the pain stabbed through her foot with each step. It hurt so bad she had to fight back tears. Kat fell back and helped her along. They kept a good pace, but it was killing her. Finally, she saw the Rose Garden up ahead.

"David!" Kat called out. "Emmy's got a blister."

"Sit down in the grass," he said.

"I'm sorry! I don't know what happened!" she cried.

He grabbed his backpack and moved over to her foot. He quickly untied the laces and pulled off her shoe. Holding her foot in the air, he examined the sock.

"Nub," he said.

"What?"

"Your sock's got a nub. Must be an old one. Sometimes the fabric on an old sock gets balled up into nubs."

"Yeah," she said. "Damn! My old, reliable socks."

"Old? Yes," he replied, a twinkle in his eyes. "Reliable? Not so much. You got a spare?"

"In my backpack."

He pulled off the sock and examined the bottom of her foot very carefully, then grinned. "It's a real beauty! Wish I had my camera." Several people laughed, but Emmy just wanted to die. He saw her expression. "It'll be okay. Just relax." He pulled his blister kit from the backpack.

"What am I gonna do?" It came out as a wail. "It's at least five miles back to Aquatic Park!"

"Don't worry," he answered, his voice soothing. "You'll be fine. You can go around the Pacific hill." He pulled out a single-edged razor blade. "Kat, would you hold her foot?" Moving around beside him, Kat lifted it up so he had a good angle. "This is gonna hurt, so you'd may as well grit your teeth."

Without further warning, he sliced right through the blister. Gasping, she held her breath, but felt amazing relief as the fluid ran out. As Kat held her foot, he deftly sliced away the dead skin. Wiping the razor, he put it back in his kit. After dabbing the wound with gauze to dry it, he rubbed some Neosporin on the tender area. It felt cool and soothing. She watched as he cut moleskin and applied it to her foot. He wrapped gauze around the wound, then, taking a wide roll of medical tape, he wrapped it round and round to hold the bandage in place.

"There," he said. "Good as new. Neosporin morning and night. Fresh bandages every day. Give it air Wednesday through Friday, in the evening. You'd better skip next Saturday's walk. Give it air all day Saturday and you should be fine by Sunday for Bay to Breakers."

He was so calm that she couldn't help but feel better. And she really didn't want to miss Bay To Breakers.

Removing fresh socks from the Whale, she sprinkled the inside of each with baby powder, then slipped them on. She put on her shoes and tightened the laces, then stood up. To test it, she rocked the foot back and forth. It felt good. She pushed off and there was pain, but nothing like she'd felt a few minutes earlier. David was—once again—right. She should be okay.

Glancing at his wrist watch, David looked around. "We're on the clock, people. Let's get moving."

They continued through the park. It hurt when she used her normal stride, so she took shorter steps and the pain was quite bearable. She didn't even lose much speed, but exhaustion was taking its toll. Twenty-three miles was indeed a real kick in the butt. Her hip joints were swollen and her back ached. They emerged from the park and headed north toward California Pacific.

After the break, Emmy left the others and took the short hill to Lyons and Pacific. She slowed down and arrived just as the team finished the hill. They now had less than two miles to go and it was all flat or downhill. Try as she may, she fell further behind the group. Bertina slowed down and walked beside her.

"Thanks for walking with me," Emmy said.

"It's okay," Bertina answered. "Honestly, I hurt so bad I can't go any faster."

"Well, you should be really proud. I hate to say it, but back when you started, I didn't think you'd make it."

"Me neither. I may not make it yet."

"You'll make it."

Bertina's silence was unsettling. Something was working on her. Emmy saw that she was hurting from more than just the day's walk. They eased themselves down Franklin until they hit a red light. Bertina was completely lost in thought, so Emmy turned to her.

"What is it?" she asked. "Something's wrong."

Bertina looked at her, eyes daring and desperate. "Don't tell anybody. I need your promise not to tell *anybody* on the team."

Out of nowhere, a gigantic lump pressed against Emmy's throat. *Please don't let it be breast cancer! Please, please!*

"Okay," she answered, swallowing. "I promise."

"I can't raise enough money. I got fourteen hundred, but I got nobody left to ask."

Relief flooded through her. *Thank God!*

Bertina's problem actually had a cure. And she could help. It hurt more to limp across the street than to drum up five hundred dollars. Her brain was pretty fried, but she knew she could think of something.

"All your letters are out?"

"Yes."

"Did you try Mayor Willie?"

"Willie Brown? Why would I try him?"

"Well, he's a liberal—he *should* support the 3-Day. I'm sure if you word the letter just right, he'll help. Try state senators, city council, and the governor. Businesses in your neighborhood. You should try. Someone'll come through. You'll see."

"Okay, I'll try."

"I've still got checks coming in. I could pass 'em on."

Bertina shook her head. "I won't take your donations. If I walk, it's got to be on *my* terms, from *my* work."

"Okay, but try Mayor Willie."

For the first time, Bertina smiled. "Thanks."

At ten minutes after twelve, they finally approached Aquatic Park. Bertina went directly to the bus stop, but Emmy limped on down to the benches. She was so burned out, she couldn't even think any more. Hobbling to a vacant bench, she sat.

David strolled over. "How are you?"

"I hurt. Everywhere."

He sat next to her. "That probably wasn't as easy as I made it out to be, but you've proved you're strong, Emmy, a lot stronger than you think."

"Thanks for taking care of me."

"Glad to do it." He smiled, then, rising, he shouldered his backpack. "See you next Sunday. Oh, don't forget your 3-Day tee shirt. We'll all be wearing them."

"I won't forget."

He tightened his backpack and walked resolutely up Van Ness Avenue. She shook her head. He truly astounded her.

How many miles can he walk in one day?

"You're crazy, David!"

Turning with a little smile, he disappeared up the street.

She looked around for Ross, but there was no sign of him. Forcing herself to move, she dug out her cell, limped down the sidewalk and speed-dialed his number.

"Hello?" he answered.

"It's me."

"Hey, Emmy, what's up?"

What was he thinking? It was like she'd called him at work or something.

"What's up? We're done. It's after noon."

"After noon? Damn! I'm sorry. I lost track of the time. I'll be right there."

"Okay." She was too exhausted to put up a fuss. In fact, she was really grateful he was coming. "Thanks, Ross," she said. "I really appreciate it."

He was silent for a moment. "Are you okay?"

"I got a blister. It was a hard walk."

"Just stay put. I'll be right there."

When she pushed the End button, she breathed out. Drifting back, she sat down again. Kat gathered up her gear.

"Need a ride?"

"No," Emmy answered. "Thanks. Ross is coming."

"Okay." She rubbed Emmy's shoulder. "You did great today." Emmy sighed and shook her head. "Come on!" Kat said. "You walked five miles on a blister. Give yourself *some* credit. You did great!"

Emmy smiled up at her. "Thanks."

With mincing steps, Kat walked across to her Honda, moving slowly, like an old lady. It gave Emmy some measure of comfort that the walk had kicked Kat's butt, too. The Honda pulled out of the lot. Sitting alone on the bench, Emmy watched tourists wandering by and runners and bicycles moving swiftly up and down the path to Fort Mason. It seemed like forever since her nightmare.

She closed her eyes.

All she wanted was to sleep.

The movement around her settled into a gentle buzz of sound. Just as she started to doze, she heard a car door close. She opened her eyes and there was Ross, standing by the car. It made her feel so good, she grinned like an idiot. He grinned right back and there was something in his eyes she'd never seen before. Something was different.

She forced herself up and hobbled toward him. Quickly, he put an arm around her and helped her along, opening the door and scooping her into the seat. She'd never felt so tired in her entire life.

As he made the turnaround and headed back up Van Ness, she looked over at him.

"I'm sorry."

He glanced at her. "For what?"

"For anything I did... or said... to hurt you or piss you off. I'm so sorry."

When he glanced back at her again, he was smiling.

"It's okay," he answered. "I love you."

Famous last words.

20

Her body jumped and for a moment, she was paralyzed with fear. Where was she? She was still in her walking gear, but in a darkened room. *Oh, yeah!* She had taken a couple of Motrin. *No wonder.* It was Ross's bed.

Everything was fuzzy and her mouth was totally dry. She didn't want to move. Every time she shifted a little, it hurt, but she had to pee, so there was no choice. Pushing herself up on her elbows, she saw the shades were drawn. She ran her tongue around the inside of her mouth, trying to wet it.

As she pushed herself up to sit, pain shot from her back down to her feet. She saw her bandaged foot in the dim light and it all came rushing back. She had a blister! *Damn it!*

Flexing her legs against the stiffness, she pushed herself out of bed and stood up. As her weight came down on her ankles, they both cracked. She pushed off on her right foot, but stopped immediately, gasping and clenching her teeth to keep from crying out. Using her heel, she hobbled into the bathroom. She didn't want to shower with her foot bandaged, so she undressed and washed up at the sink—as much as she hurt, it was an Olympic feat. She brushed her teeth so her mouth felt clean, then slipped on her robe and limped back to the bedroom.

Ross stuck his head in.

"Hey, babe. How you doing?"

"Other than being crippled?"

"Other than being crippled..."

"Not bad." She yawned. "How long did I sleep?" *I know I have clean clothes here somewhere.*

"Almost four hours," he answered. "You needed it." He stepped behind her at the dresser and slipped his arms around her belly. Gently, he kissed her neck. "I thought we might order in tonight."

"I'm starving," she said, leaning back into him.

"What do you want? Chinese? Pizza?"

"I think I deserve pizza."

"Okay," he said, kissing her head. "You get dressed. I'll get something ordered."

Dressing was a challenge, but eventually she hobbled out into the living room just as the pizza arrived.

"Okay," he said, bringing plates from the kitchen, "how'd you get the blister?"

She pulled a slice of pizza from the box and plunked it on her plate. "It was stupid. One of my old socks had a nub in it that rubbed against the ball of my foot."

It started a series of questions that he asked continually as they ate. It was a little confusing. He hadn't shown any interest before, but now he wanted to know everything. Especially, he wanted to know about the people she trained with, so she told him about David and the others.

"So, this David bandaged your foot?" he asked.

"It was amazing. He did the whole thing in about a minute. I was afraid I couldn't get back, but he said I'd make it and I did. I trust him, Ross. He's a good man."

He nodded. "I'm glad you're with good people."

"Listen," she said, "I meant what I said. I'm really sorry."

Pushing his plate aside, he faced her. "Me, too. Maybe all of this work raising money to fight cancer hits a little too close to home."

She hadn't thought of that. *Stupid.* She rested her hand on his knee. "I've decided that part's over. We've sent out the last of the letters. There's just one more thing I want to do and it won't involve you at all."

"What's that?"

"Bake sale with Mom and Grace."

He smiled. "Well, I wouldn't be any good at that."

"So—is there anything else on your mind?"

"I don't know," he said. "It seems like we're just not having any fun. When we first got together we were always laughing and goofing around. Now, it's just all serious."

It was time to tell him. She had to tell him about herself, but she wasn't sure how to come clean. She swallowed.

Just tell him.

"There's something I haven't told you about." She took a deep breath and blew it out. "I.. uh... I've been fighting depression... for a long time now—about five years, but since Amy died, it's been worse." He nodded, as if he might understand. "In fact—"

She couldn't go on.

He leaned over and took her hands in his.

"It's okay, Emmy. You can tell me anything."

She wasn't sure about that. She was afraid of his reaction, so she squeezed his hands.

"I took a bottle of pills. You know?" He nodded again. "Not enough. Didn't work. Mom put me in therapy. I'm still there."

She blew out a long breath and looked up into his eyes.

"I'm sorry," he said. "I hope you don't feel like you could do something like that now?"

"No! I'm getting better. Happier, I guess. Getting involved in the 3-Day really helped. *You've* helped. You've helped a lot. We'll have more fun together, I promise."

Leaning over, he kissed her quickly, softly.

"I'll do whatever I can."

"Just be yourself."

They looked into each other's eyes. Things had changed. It felt good to open up to him. Maybe she had matured a little. She still hadn't told him about how messed up her family was—or the whole obsessive-compulsive issue, but she would tell him. *I know I will.*

He picked up their plates and took them into the kitchen. She leaned back on the sofa to watch him. "I had an idea today." He stopped. "I can drive. If you'll loan me the car, you can sleep in. How's that sound?"

Turning around, he smiled sheepishly. "I'd like that."

"I thought you might..."

He leaned back against the sink and looked at her.

"I owe you an apology, too. For the banana and for getting mad at you. I'm sorry. I guess I have some problems, too."

"It's okay. We'll be okay."

Smiling, he turned back to the sink. While he rinsed the dishes, she called her mother to work out details of the bake sale. It would be on the last weekend of the month. She would skip training, but do flat walks in Pleasanton to make it up.

As she wrapped up the call, Ross leaned down and peeked inside the Whale. He pulled out the 3-Day book, leafed through it, then started to type on his computer. She disconnected and watched Ross for a moment. It was already time to go home.

She hobbled up behind him. "What are you doing?"

"Oh, just making a few notes."

"About the 3-Day?"

"Uh huh."

"How come?"

"I got an idea this afternoon," he answered, swiveling around to face her. He rested his hands on her hips and leaned forward to kiss her stomach.

"What kind of idea?"

He looked up into her eyes.

"I want to write about the Walk."

"Really? What are you gonna write?"

"I don't know," he answered, "but when I pulled up in the car this afternoon and saw you sitting on the bench... you looked... battered." He paused for a moment, gathering his words. "What you're doing is amazing. All I know right now is that I want to learn as much as I can. I'll figure out what to do with it later."

"That's pretty cool," she said. "People should know about it. I hate to bring this up, but I have to go home."

"Stay," he said. "Stay the whole week. It's gonna be hard enough getting that foot healed without walking back and forth to the bus stop. I can drive you in and bring you home. If you need more clothing, we'll go over and get it."

It *would* be a busy week. She had to pick up her memorial shirt from the print shop. She was meeting with Dan Fleming on Tuesday to pass it along to him so that he could sign it and get Annie and Ben's signatures. That would be hard enough.

She looked into his eyes. "Thank you, Ross. For everything."

He nodded, smiling, and held her close.

Things were getting better already.

21

Tuesday, May 15

"Have a seat, he'll be with you in a minute."

Turning, Emmy limped over to the waiting area. She dropped her carryall and the plastic bag on a leather sofa and sat. The office was ten times more luxurious than Markham Graphics. She felt glad she'd worn a nice outfit. The only thing that didn't fit was her running shoes, but she had to wear the softer shoes because of her bandaged foot.

She was so glad Ross had put her up for the week. Her foot was healing really fast. Hopefully, it would be good on Sunday. And hopefully she wouldn't gain much weight. She'd been lunching with Tina and Joanna and was scheduled for lunch with Kat on Friday.

Whatever Ross had seen at Aquatic Park last Sunday had really charged him up. They talked about the Walk a lot now—and now he seemed to be excited about meeting her family, too.

She'd decided that regardless of how much money the bake sale brought in, she was going to share it with Bertina. She had decided to donate it anonymously. It meant a lot to have Bertina walk with them—it was worth risking her friendship.

A door down the hall opened and Dan appeared.

"Emmy!" he called as he approached her. "It's so good to see you again!"

"You, too!"

He hugged her and just the smell of him brought back good memories. She picked up her stuff and he turned to lead her to his office, but when she stepped out, she had to limp.

"You okay?" he asked, slowing down to walk beside her.

"Yeah. I got a stupid blister last weekend."

"Training?" She nodded. "How's it going?"

"Good," she answered. "We did our first twenty-three mile walk on Sunday. That's where I got the blister."

"Well, you look terrific. You've lost so much weight!"

"Thanks!"

She was glad he'd noticed. It was kind of a stupid secret thrill, but it really meant a lot. They entered his office, which was nearly twice as large as Jack Markham's. His work was spread out across the room in little stacks. Following him to a casual area, she sat down on the sofa and he sat in a chair next to her by the coffee table.

"How is everything?" she asked. "It's been a while."

"Things are okay," he answered. "Not the same, of course, but we're getting by. Annie and Ben are busy with school. The anniversary was hard, but we got through it."

"I'm glad."

"Twenty-three miles," he repeated, shaking his head. "You said this is the *first* twenty-three mile walk?"

"Yeah, we'll walk it four times altogether, including a simulation of all three days. I'm training with a really good group. I'll be ready by July. Believe it or not, I've raised almost forty-three hundred dollars."

A surprised smile spread across his face.

"Emmy, that's wonderful! I bet that's why you're here," he said, reaching into his suit coat and pulling out a checkbook.

"No! No. I'm not asking for a donation. I'm here for something else."

He hesitated, then smiled again. "Well, I hope you'll accept a donation if I give it?"

She looked into his eyes. "I wouldn't turn it down, but it's not why I'm here."

"Why *did* you come?"

"I have a favor to ask." This was it. Swallowing, she reached down, lifted the plastic bag from the carpet and pulled out her memorial tee shirt. "I brought something to show you." As she held it up, he saw the black lettering on the front:

AMELIA FLEMING

October 20, 1959—April 16, 2000

She closed her eyes so she didn't have to look at the back, then turned the shirt around so he could see the large photo of Amy at her birthday party, flashing a beautiful smile, her eyes bright. He took it from her hands and stared at it for a long moment, his eyes glinting with tears. She swallowed against the lump in her throat and worked to find her voice.

"I'll wear this on Day Two," she said. "I was wondering if you would take it home and if you and Annie and Ben would sign it for me." She pulled a black pen from the bag. "I brought a Sharpie for you. It would mean a lot if the three of you signed it."

He dropped the shirt to his lap and looked at her, his eyes still glistening. "And I thought you were coming for money," he said, his voice choking. "God, I'm so sorry, Emmy."

"It's okay," she answered, squeezing his hand.

"Of course we'll sign it!" Holding up the shirt again, he stared at the picture. "She was so beautiful."

Emmy nodded, fearing for her voice.

He cleared his throat, but didn't say anything. When she lifted the bag, he passed the shirt back to her. It was a relief to fold it up. She put it back in the bag with the Sharpie and set it on the table for him. For a moment, he seemed lost in thought, almost as if fighting with himself, then swiftly he found a pen and opened his checkbook.

"Who does it get made out to?"

"Avon Breast Cancer 3-Day."

He wrote the check quickly, ripped it out and passed it over. The second she looked at it, she knew she couldn't accept it.

"Dan, this is too much. You can't—"

"I can," he said, smiling. "I have."

It was easy to see why Amy had loved him so much. Her throat swelled. *I can't cry. I won't let myself cry.* She shook her head.

"Listen to me." He leaned closer, his eyes intent. She looked up at him. "The only real value money has is what we do with it. I want this money to mean something. I want it to work for something more valuable than that little scrip of paper. You're doing something wonderful here, Emmy. Let me do my part to help find a cure."

She felt unable to speak, so she simply nodded.

22

Training Journal of Emmy Wells

5/15	Tuesday	Rest. Lunch with Kat.
5/16	Wed.	Rest. Lunch with Ross.

Thursday, May 17, 4:37 pm

This is my fourth day of recovery from the blister. Four consecutive days with little to no walking. Man, I hope I don't lose much conditioning. David said I should be okay, so I should be okay.

The check from Dan Fleming is propped against my keyboard.

I always took him for granted. Aunt Amy always deserved the best, but before him she went through a string of weird guys. Then she married an asshole and it screwed up her life for another five years. And when that was over—when she was alone again—she did her very best work, passionate and powerful. That's when she took me under her wing and I adopted her, but every time Mom dropped me off at the studio, I saw how lonely Amy was. Maybe that sparked her work. She was missing something.

Then, one day, Dan showed up and he was missing something, too, so they found each other. Dan's the whole package: wealthy, handsome, a passionate collector of fine art. I think he truly understood her. I've always been a little jealous, but he's a good man and I have to admit that he was perfect for her.

It was a shock when she moved to San Francisco after they were married, but I still saw her a lot. Then she got breast cancer and everything was crazy. Dan thought it would be best if they moved her studio to a more secluded location—far enough away that she could work in peace without constant demands on her time.

So they bought the ranch with the lake.

And she was gone. Just like that.

I wish I would have appreciated him more in happier days. He *is* a good man and they *were* perfect together.

How can I give away his donation?

And yet here I am. I just can't ignore the symmetry. Bertina is five hundred dollars short and I have a five hundred dollar check. It was meant to happen this way. It all goes for the same thing.

I've printed out a copy of Bertina's donation form and I've filled it in. Donor's name: Anonymous. Amount: $500.00.

So why do I feel awful?

I'm off work in a few minutes and I'm going to take it over to the 3-Day office. They'll process it without any questions.

And I'll be done.

I only hope Bertina doesn't find out it was me.

23

Sunday, May 20

As she crossed Lombard in the Scoupe, she was only sure of one thing—she'd be walking again. And it was going to be a fun walk this time. Every year, the City celebrated Bay to Breakers and yet Emmy had never even watched. Although it was technically a race, only a few runners cared about that part. It was really just a gigantic parade—one big twelve kilometer party—east to west—all the way across San Francisco to the Pacific Ocean.

Her foot felt really good. She'd followed David's advice to the letter and it had worked. She'd rested it Saturday. In fact, they had slept until nearly ten o'clock and lazed around most of the day. She hoped it was a preview of what it would be like when the Walk was over. In the evening, they went to Ghirardelli Square for dinner at McCormick and Kuleto's and she hadn't limped at all.

She found a parking space and joined her teammates.

Everyone stretched like it was a normal training walk, but there was no sign-in sheet. Everyone was a member of the team. She found her spot next to Kat and they stretched, but she kept looking back at every new arrival.

At last, Bertina jogged up the steps. She said hi to David, then moved directly to the center to stretch. Emmy tried hard not to look at her, but she was curious if Bertina knew about the donation yet. She was excited because now Bertina could participate, but she was also afraid of being caught out. After all, Bertina had made it clear that she didn't want help. Her casual stretching revealed nothing.

"Listen up, everybody!" David stepped forward. "This isn't a normal training walk, but the rules still apply. You all know what they are. When we get to E4, make sure to use the restroom, stretch and hydrate. We need to keep together, so when we wade into the crowd, everybody keep a firm grip on the person in front of you and behind you. Don't let go until we find a good place to walk. Give your teammates a chance to work their way around knots in the crowd. If anybody gets separated, we all stop until we're together again. If anybody wants to walk back afterward, just stick with me."*

It was a very relaxed walk to the Embarcadero Center, full of chatter and laughter. It was more fun than she'd had on any walk since

---

* See Map on Page 349.

she'd started training.

Approaching E4, they waded into the crowd. Thousands of people streamed around them at a frantic pace heading south across Market Street. As they stretched, she turned to Tom and Marianne.

"How many people are in this thing?"

Tom grinned. "We set the record—what was it? 1986? A hundred twelve thousand."

"A hundred twelve thousand! Geez!"

He laughed. "Don't worry. Shouldn't be more than—oh, say eighty grand today."

"Gather round!" David called out. "Remember what I said. When we wade into the crowd, hang onto each other."

They formed their human chain immediately and David led them through the packed mass of bodies across Market Street. Even though they moved slowly, several times people broke through and they stopped, waiting to reform the chain.

Shouts, laughter, the chatter of so many people talking, and the blast of rock music through gigantic speakers created a loud, white noise all around them. Other chains of people crawled around the mass. Some people climbed lamp posts to take pictures. Tortillas flew overhead like frisbees. It was a gigantic beehive.

David found a small pocket in the mass and they reassembled, moving close together to avoid separation. At least half the crowd wore some kind of costume: everything from a five piece mariachi band to a complete brigade of male and female pirates with mustaches. A keg of beer wheeled by them driven by a band of girls wearing togas. Everywhere, the pungent smell of pot filled the air. Directly in front of them, a man and woman stood slurping margaritas from pitchers. They were painted purple from head to toe and aside from their grass skirts and running shoes, they were both completely naked.

Somewhere up ahead, a starter pistol popped, but nobody moved. Emmy waited impatiently, ready to walk.

After nearly five minutes, the people in front of them finally surged forward and Team Aquatic Park followed. She thought the team looked great, seventeen strong, all wearing their 3-Day tee shirts. It was a real log jam at first, but David moved them ahead bit by bit. About a mile into the walk, they finally had enough space to spread out.

Watching the crowd cheering them on was almost as much fun as looking at the other walkers. As they made their way through Hayes Valley, she saw an entire house that had been decorated like a cat house, complete with red lights and girls dressed in skimpy outfits leaning out the windows, waving and cheering.

Further on, the noise tapered off so they could talk without shouting back and forth. Human centipedes occasionally passed them, one in the form of a Chinese dragon and another with six runners covered in clear plastic made to look like a gigantic condom. There were more naked people than she'd expected, some running and some just flashing the crowd. Almost all of them were covered in body paint and that seemed to be a very good thing.

The time passed quickly and before she was quite aware of it, they had walked completely across the City. She was surprised at how easy it was. Of course, there was only one small hill on the route—that made a *big* difference. By the time they had checked into the party area at Golden Gate Park, a band was playing and people were dancing.

Settling into a quiet area, they stretched for a while, then most of the others went off to join the party. Tom's wife showed up and they wandered off to have fun. As Emmy had hoped, the group had shrunk down to two: she and David. He tightened his fanny pack (his own Minnow, matching hers) and they began walking back across the City.

As if by habit, they headed straight toward the California Pacific Medical Center, chatting about the Bay to Breakers. After a while, they walked in silence, then David turned his head to her.

"So, are you in school?" he asked.

"Mornings. Afternoons I work for a graphic design company in Embarcadero Two."

"So we cover your stomping grounds a lot."

"Well, I never take the stairs the way we do," she answered with a small chuckle. "What do you do?"

"I'm an Office Manager," he replied. "Pretty dry job. Handle personnel decisions, arbitrate disputes, do employee reviews. Order office supplies. That sort of thing. You wouldn't know me in a business suit."

"Are you from San Francisco?"

"Born and raised. What about you?"

"Pleasanton."

"Nice little city."

"Yes," she agreed.

As they approached the medical center, he glanced at her. "I'm really sorry about your aunt."

"Thanks." She shrugged, looking down at the sidewalk. From the corner of her eye, she saw his face slant in a funny sort of look, but when she turned her head to him, he glanced down the block.

After using the restrooms, they met out front and sat on the bench at the end of the little path, taking fluids. It was the first time she'd been alone with him and the perfect time to ask her question. If she didn't ask him now, she might never get the chance.

"It's none of my business," she said, "and you don't have to talk about it if you don't want to, but... you said you lost someone here, too." He didn't say anything, so she pressed on. "I was wondering who it was."

He sat in silence, unmoving. After a few moments of thought, he took off his glasses and held them in his hand.

"Joey." He spoke softly. "I lost Joanna here."

She must have been his wife. Emmy couldn't stop herself from asking it aloud.

"Your wife?"

He nodded his head slowly, then turned to face her.

"Sometimes you get lucky in life and I got lucky with her. She had something special. There's never been anybody like her." He was silent again, looking down at the sidewalk. "I thought she was crazy when she hooked up with me. I mean, who am I? She could have had anybody, but she chose me. I'd do anything for her, anything at all, but when she needed me the most, I couldn't help." He glanced at the building, then stared out at the street. "I couldn't do a damned thing."

Sighing, he slipped his glasses back on.

The silence stretched out between them, then Emmy put her hand on his shoulder and rubbed it, just like Marianne had done for her. When he turned to look at her, she smiled at him.

"I know why she picked you."

With a look of surprise, he cocked his head to the side and waited for her to continue.

"You're a special person, David. You love these walkers, you work with everybody to make them better walkers, to make sure they do good. I've never seen anybody as dedicated to one thing. You take care of us all."

He cleared his throat and stood up. It was hard to read his expression, but she knew that she'd touched him. They walked out onto the grass along the steps.

"I've *got* to look after everybody," he said, deadpan. "Without me, half these people would be dead." A small smile tugged at the corner of his mouth. "Including you."

He bent down to stretch and Emmy laughed.

It was pure David and she loved him for it.

24

Training Calendar of Team Aquatic Park

6/17	Sunday	23 Mile Hill Walk.
6/23	Saturday	18 Mile Hill Walk.
6/24	Sunday	10 Mile Fun Walk Sausalito.*

Sunday, June 24, 4:35 pm

What an amazing day!

Today was our ten mile fun walk to Sausalito and it was truly astounding, although it did start out with a bummer. Ross gave me a ride to Aquatic Park since we didn't start until 8 am. On the way, he told me that during his visit to the 3-Day office—he's still researching the whole 3-Day thing—he found out that not *all* of our donations go to fight breast cancer!

What a shocker!

I always thought that Avon paid for it—lots of free advertising,

---

*See Map on Page 327.

good will. No. Avon and Pallotta have a partnership and a big percentage of the money raised goes to pay Pallotta's expenses.

Ross said it varies from one event to another and there are nine events this year across the country. The percentage depends on what each one costs and how much money they bring in. Every location is a little different.

I feel like such a dummy, thinking all the money goes directly to fight cancer when it looks like a big amount is diverted.

How much?

I wonder if David knows—I wonder what he thinks.

We should find out soon because I introduced Ross to him and they set up an interview. Ross originally wanted the interview just for a profile, but now the Pallotta question is tops in my mind. I really want to know.

Anyway, I got the introductions done and Ross spent all the time while we were warming up talking to people like Marianne and Joy and Ellen. After that, he went back home to type up his notes. We had planned for him to meet me in Sausalito so we could look at some houses and apartments over there.

Kat was right up in my grill about how serious we're getting and plainly asked if we had set a date!

Man, that's crazy! I mean, we're not even anywhere close to thinking about marriage. Hell, I'm not even sure we can live together yet. I do spend a lot of time at his place, but it's still not like seeing him day in and day out. I may hate it. I don't know!

But it really set off Michael and Tom.

Michael said, "I can't wait till Kat gets married! I'm sure she'll fall in love with Mr. Thomas Nip, then she'll be *Kat Nip*!"

It was so funny! Kat just rolled her eyes. Then Tom said, "No, she's gonna fall in love with Mr. Bill Chup, then she'll be *Kat Chup*!"

I couldn't tell if Kat was pissed or not, but she kind of growled and said, "You're both wrong. I'm gonna marry Mr. Jim House and then I'll be "*Kat House*!"

All three of them said it together and it was so funny I almost peed myself laughing.

Anyway, we went on the Northern route. I love the northern route. It goes right up to Fort Point, then up to the Golden Gate Bridge Toll Plaza.

The pace today was quite leisurely for us. It was fun, just as advertised. And just the team.

I walked up front with David, Kat, Tom, Marianne, and the others. Lauren was right behind, with Alex and Darla. At the crest of Fort Mason, I looked across the Bay to Sausalito. It sits on the lee of the Marin Headlands and it's truly a beautiful city.

Along the Marina Green, David pointed out where the stage will be set up for the Closing Ceremony, the final stop of our three days of walking.

Continuing on to Crissy Field, we crossed over to a path that leads along the beach. Lazy waves lapped against the shore. A girl tossed a Frisbee into the shallow water and a golden retriever bounded in after it. An elderly couple nodded to us as we passed. It was a just a glorious day!

I don't know why, but today I just felt so alive. The breeze was chill and fresh. I just felt enveloped in beauty.

Then Michael starting singing "Under the Boardwalk." He has a wonderful tenor voice. Marianne joined in and pretty soon we were all singing. I've never felt more a part of a group in my life and it just feels so good to be a part of it.

I was happy. Very happy and content, but in the back of my mind, I kept thinking:

There must be something wrong.

As we approached Fort Point, I saw the underbelly of the Golden Gate Bridge—the long, rust-red tubes that hold the gigantic suspension cables. They arch out of the headlands and soar up to the heights of the towers. You never realize how big they are until you're standing under them.

We cut over to the long switchback road that leads up to the Toll Plaza and when we got there, it was still warm and sunny.

It was so warm I thought maybe I didn't need my thermals. Marianne and Tom put the lid on that. Tom even said Ripley's "Believe It or Not" was opening a display of frozen Golden Gate Bridge tourists down on Fisherman's Wharf.

So I put on my thermals, then my windbreaker. We had a good stretch, then headed up the walkway to the bridge. Immediately, the stiff, icy wind blasted through me. Gusts grabbed at my arms, inflating the windbreaker. We eased our way toward the center and the wind died away enough to stop and take photos with Alcatraz and Angel Island behind us.

As I looked across the Bay, I felt chills, literally, but not from the wind. Looking at the dark green parkland of the Presidio, bulking up on my right, sweeping from the headlands east to the skyline of buildings downtown, with the Transamerica Pyramid needling up and Coit Tower rising on Telegraph Hill, all the way across the City to the Bay Bridge and beyond to Berkeley and Oakland, I just felt stunned with the beauty.

My heart pounded—it pounds now just thinking about it. I knew then there wasn't any point in looking at rentals in Sausalito. I'll never leave the City. David's routes have opened up San Francisco to me in a way few people will ever know. It's so much more than tall buildings and busy streets. The hills and parks and woodlands make a Garden of Eden if you know where to go.

And I do.

I'm blessed to be here, to be a part of this, and to be among the most wonderful people I've ever known.

San Francisco is my home now.

I'll never leave.

25

Training Calendar of Emmy Wells

6/27	Wed.	3 Miles Embarcadero, Pier 39.
6/28	Thursday	3 Miles, Embarcadero, Pier 39.

Friday, June 29

Sim—Day 1

"I know you're tired," Ross said as he drove toward Aquatic Park in the early morning traffic, "but if you think of it, please confirm tomorrow's interview with David."

"Okay."

She sat immovable, burned out. Having awakened a little after two o'clock in the morning and unable to return to sleep, she felt lost and groggy, but totally committed to the next three days of walking.

I can make it. I know I can.

The Sim. *Geez!* Fifty-nine miles over three days, including the roughest part—twenty-three miles—on this morning when she was burned out and exhausted. But she had to do it. Another yawn. The weekends had piled up on her, mile after relentless mile. Thirteen. Eighteen. Twenty. Twenty three. Again. According to her Training Journal, she had walked over eight hundred miles so far and she felt every one of them.

It was a Friday morning—a work day—and the streets were clogged with rush hour traffic. She couldn't figure out why David was starting at eight o'clock instead five. They would be smack in the middle of traffic and wouldn't get back until at least three o'clock. It would be hard enough walking twenty-three miles, but in the middle of work-day traffic? *It just doesn't make sense!*

Of course, it didn't make sense to be there at all. She was missing school and work and she felt guilty about both, but the Sim was extremely important. Once she'd done it, she knew she could do the real thing. It was that third day. How would she hold up when push came to shove? This twenty-three miles would prove a lot, but she had to fight through the exhaustion. She had to do it.

Ross pulled into an empty parking space. She reached for the Whale, but he gently touched her arm.

"Wish I could pick you up," he said.

"I'm okay with the bus. I'll just see you tonight." She leaned over to kiss him. "Thanks for the ride."

When she arrived at the bleachers, no one else was there, so she sat down and closed her eyes. *I'd give anything to go back to bed.* Within a minute, David trotted up the stairs.

"Hey, Emmy! You're early."

"Hey, David. Ross dropped me off on his way to work."

"You ready?"

"We'll see. We still on for the interview?"

"Sure, three o'clock tomorrow. I'll be there."

She'd been really looking forward to it. This whole thing about a percentage of the funds going to Pallotta seriously bothered her. It seemed like—well, they didn't exactly lie, but it seemed like a big sin of omission. It should have been out front. The big question was: how much? *What's the percentage?*

It was a small group, mostly team members, but with a few others Emmy didn't know. Tom and Michael were missing, but it was a Friday, so she felt lucky that anybody had made it. Kat and Marianne both took the day off from work and Emmy was very happy they were there. So were Karen and Rhonda. And she was relieved that Juliette made it before David started the briefing. There were fifteen walkers, including David.

A teenager, short and thin, with wavy black hair and keen black eyes, moved down to stretch alongside Kat and Emmy.

"Hi," she said, "I'm Rachel Timmons."

Timmons? It rang a bell—not exactly a common name. Then it hit her: *Jessica Timmons! Tom's patient!* Could this be her daughter? Unconsciously, she glanced around, but Tom wasn't there, so she turned her attention back to Rachel.

"Emmy Wells."

Kat introduced herself, then Marianne joined them a moment later. Rachel had been training on Mount Diablo and that was quite impressive. Glancing at her legs, Emmy figured she would be able to hold her own on the hills.

David passed out six maps, which wasn't a good sign.* She thought that Rachel would be okay, but worried that the other newcomers wouldn't keep the pace. It would be hard enough without having people scattered all over the City.

"Welcome to Day One," David said. "Today, we're walking twenty-three miles. We're starting at eight o'clock because Day One

---

See Map on Page 355.

will start around then and this will simulate the conditions. You can't believe how hard it'll be to make your way through two thousand walkers. The foot traffic we'll face this morning will give you a small taste. There's also a lot of traffic lights on Day One and we'll get our share today. Lots of stop and start, so stay loose. Don't let your legs tighten up waiting for a light to change."

Emmy was stunned. He had done it on purpose—making it hard and long and ugly, just so they would get a taste of how it was on Day One. She felt so burned out that his announcement made her think once again about quitting.

It would be sheer hell and she just felt dead.

They made their way toward Fisherman's Wharf, ambling along at three miles an hour; they couldn't go any faster, dodging and ducking vendors and tourists. Past Pier 39, the pace picked up and it felt good, but there were people everywhere.

At the Embarcadero Center, Kat ran up and down each stairwell, but Emmy merely pegged along. On the Clay Street hill, dodging pedestrians became a nightmare. They were stopped at nearly every light in Chinatown. Sometimes it was impossible to pass people. Doing the hill in slow motion hurt and each step pissed her off more and more.

Why am I doing this?

How about an exit plan?

At Lafayette Park, she could duck out, go to Ross's apartment and crash. All she wanted was to lie down and sleep. He'd never know. She glanced at Kat. *She'd know.* Everyone on the team would know. They topped the Clay Street hill and were into the residential area with less foot traffic and practically no stoplights. David kicked it into gear and she began to relax. It felt great to stretch it out.

I can do this. I know I can do this. I just have to hang in.

At Lafayette Park, David waited for the slow walkers to catch up. Instead of having someone lead the slower walkers, he had kept the whole group together. Probably because there were so few people on the walk, but it pissed her off anyway. She had to move just to stay awake.

Turning to Kat, she mumbled, "I hate waiting around. I want to get moving!" Marianne stopped stretching. Looking perturbed, she glanced at Emmy, then turned away.

They moved at a steady pace all the way to California Pacific and Emmy found her zone again. Even the slower walkers did well with no hills to impede their progress. It was a pretty good break, but she kept checking her watch, waiting, waiting. They lost more time on the detour through the Presidio. David halted everyone at the top of the hill, so the slower walkers could catch up.

Emmy walked around in a circle, cursing softly as she paced.

When they finally got to Mountain Lake, she felt totally spent and they weren't even half way through. Sitting on a bench, she stretched her tight legs. They were much stiffer than usual and it really bothered her. She glanced at her wristwatch.

God! It's almost noon!

She turned to Marianne and Kat.

"Geez, this is frustrating!"

Marianne stood and fixed her with a piercing stare.

"You know, Emmy, you're starting to piss me off. There's nothing we can do about it, okay? There are some things in life we just can't do anything about." She stopped her tirade and stared at Emmy. "Look, either you can suck it up and try to make the best of it or you can shut up and not make it worse for the rest of us."

Emmy stood in shock. It was like Marianne had just slapped her across the face. She tingled all over and flushed. Blood pounded in her ears. Marianne just called her out for bitching—in front of the whole team. It was humiliating.

Was I really that bitchy?

Oh, shit! I was.

She'd let her frustration boil over. The last thing she wanted was to alienate Marianne, a woman she truly and deeply respected. Tears came to her eyes, but she blinked them away. Somehow, she had to suck it up, to make the best of a bad situation.

And for God's sake, shut up. Just shut up, Emmy, okay?

The break was over and she expended her new humiliation energy on the long trek to Cliff House. They were moving fast now and the speed was a tonic. She fell into an incredible rhythm, her entire body tingling with the exertion. Everything worked together in harmony. She would make things right with Marianne. She *had* to. Somehow, she would be a better person. Lost inside her stride, she felt like she could walk forever. After almost four miles of being alone in herself, she crested the final hill and faced the ocean.

Once again, at Cliff House, she had to wait around, but she knew she had to be patient. She kept her mouth shut and went about her business calmly. First, she powdered her feet and changed socks. After the blister incident, she always changed socks at Cliff House.

Her stomach groaned. She was starving and she was sick of trail mix. If she had to wait, she was going to take a lunch break and rest. Reluctantly, she stepped up to the hot dog vendor and ordered. Before she could even squiggle mustard on the dog, Kat, Karen, and Rhonda were in line behind her.

Although she didn't really like hot dogs, she relished this one, gobbling it down and craving more.

It was nearly one-thirty. Dutifully, she went through her entire routine of stretches and by the time she was finished, the stragglers arrived and took their break. Emmy sat on the curb to wait. She had already stretched so much that it hurt worse than walking.

Finally, they left and once again she got a good rhythm through Golden Gate Park. Every step brought her closer to the end. She'd done the twenty-three mile walk three times now, so the stress on her body wasn't nearly as bad as it could have been, but fatigue was a different story. When they reached the Rose Garden, she threw herself down on the grass.

"Wake me up when it's time to go," she said.

"You wake *me* up," Kat answered, sprawling beside her.

They rested side by side and as Emmy dozed off she felt something tapping against the bottom of her foot. She opened her eyes to see David standing over them, gently kicking first her left foot and then Kat's right.

"Enough already!" Kat growled. "I get the point."

Helping each other, they pulled themselves up. Emmy glanced at the path as two of the late walkers, older women, hobbled into the break area and threw themselves on the grass near Emmy and Kat. These ladies faced more than just fatigue. They hurt bad and it was getting worse with each passing mile.

"Hang in there," Emmy said. "Next time, it'll be a lot easier."

David encouraged everyone to stretch and hydrate, so Emmy did both. Before they left, she gave each of the older women a few Motrin to help with the pain.

As they continued through the park and then north, she walked along in a daze, so tired she hardly noticed when they approached the medical center.

When she got out of the bathroom, David was working on two women who had developed blisters. She sat down and held an injured foot while David worked on it. She encouraged them by talking about her own blister and it seemed to cheer them up, at least some. David explained how to care for the wounds and they tried to be upbeat about making it back to Aquatic Park.

"Listen up, everybody," David said. "I'm gonna help these two up California and Lyon so they don't have to do the hill. If anybody wants to come with us, you're welcome."

"I'm on the hill," Marianne said immediately. "Who's with me?" She looked around at the team expectantly.

Emmy stepped forward, looking her in the eye, then Kat stepped up beside her with a weary smile.

"It wouldn't seem like a training walk," she said, "if we left the cherry off the top."

Quickly, Karen, Rhonda, and Juliette joined them. Rachel Timmons flashed a smile and nodded her head.

"I'm in," she said.

I like this girl.

The other walkers went with David.

Although the Pacific hill wasn't as menacing as it used to be, it was, nonetheless, still quite difficult at the end of any walk. Emmy stood at the bottom looking up at it. Why was she doing it today? Her calves and feet ached and she was dead tired, but somehow she put one foot in front of the other and steadily worked her way up it. Staying right behind Marianne every step of the way, she worked on her breathing, in time with her footwork, and ground it out.

When she stood at the top, she blew out a deep breath. Looking down at the other five walkers behind her, she knew why she had to do it. Taking this ugly hill, toward the end of twenty-three miles, was a real achievement. She didn't know what it meant to anybody else, but for Emmy Wells, this was the new life, the life she planned to lead.

Marianne tapped her arm and pointed down Lyon Street. David led a MASH unit up the little hill, with several tired walkers helping to support the ladies with blisters. It was already three-twenty, but that didn't matter any more.

She looked into Marianne's eyes.

"I'm sorry," she said.

Marianne turned on her beautiful smile.

"It's okay," she answered. "If I hadn't been so pissed off myself, I probably wouldn't have dumped on you. Friends?"

She offered her hand and Emmy shook it.

"Friends."

The group reassembled and set off for the final two miles. When they arrived at Aquatic Park, she was completely beat. All she wanted to do was go to bed. Her hip joints were swollen, her calves ached, and her feet felt like two useless stumps, but she knew she could gut out the pain. She would be right back here tomorrow to walk another sixteen miles and twenty more on Sunday.

A bus was scheduled to arrive at four-twenty and she was determined to be on it, so she quickly stretched. It hurt, but it was necessary.

A hot shower and a cold Tsingtao.

Just get me through another hour.

At Ross's apartment, she slipped out of her stinky clothes. It hurt to lift her leg over the tub rim, but she gladly stepped into the hot water. Her hair was salty and her scalp scaly. She worked the shampoo into mountainous suds. She scrubbed until she was completely clean, then rinsed and stood under the spray until the water ran tepid.

She stepped up to the mirror and it was like looking at herself for the first time. Her face had lost its roundness. Her waist and belly were slim and her hips were tight. How could this possibly be Emmy Wells?

One thing was certain: she would never stop walking or go back to the way she had been. She would walk year round, by herself, with her friends, and in marathons and fundraising events. But from January to July of every year, she would train with the team and raise money to end breast cancer.

To end breast cancer.

It never meant much to her before. She signed up for the Walk because Barb and Tina encouraged her to do it, but as the days passed, she'd found herself longing more and more to achieve that one thing—the end of breast cancer forever. That was the real goal.

26

Saturday, June 30

Sim—Day 2 *

"There's a space in that Public lot!"

It was a Chinatown lot, not far from North Beach, and they found an empty space on the third level.

She really liked Ross's car, the Scoupe, but it rode so low to the ground that it took an enormous effort to climb out with aching muscles. After walking sixteen miles—thirty-nine miles in two days—she was so sore that it hurt to turn her body. Gritting her teeth, she lifted her legs and swung them out, then used the door to haul herself out with a minimum of pain.

Thankfully, O'Reilly's wasn't far from the garage. Tables were set up on the sidewalk and the doors of the restaurant were wide open. An

---

See Map on Page 343.

Irish wolfhound lounged at the entrance, placidly watching the traffic.

David sat at the back nursing a pint of Guiness and reading. Pictures of O'Neill, Yeats and Joyce hang on the wall behind him.

It was strange to see David in a button-down shirt and jeans—and without the doo rag he wore on most of their walks. He looked good, slimmer and brighter somehow.

"Hi, David!" she called out, as they approached the table.

"Greetings," he replied, "and welcome."

They sat down across from him. A waitress delivered menus and they ordered Harp and Shepherd's Pie.

"You live in North Beach?" Ross asked.

"Russian Hill, actually, but it's fairly close. Downhill all the way here, uphill all the way home, but I really love this area. All my favorite restaurants are here."

"Kat lives on Russian Hill, too," Emmy said.

"Yeah, she's only about three blocks away from me. We get together sometimes for lunch or dinner."

She turned her head to Ross. "Maybe we should look at some places up there. We could walk to work." His face turned sour and Emmy laughed. Turning back to David, she explained, "I've been trying to get him to walk more."

David chuckled.

"Always recruiting. You guys are moving?"

"Actually, we've got our own places right now, but we're moving in together. It'll save us both a lot of money."

"No kidding."

The food arrived and they chatted about neighborhoods as they ate. "Our target date is the first of September," she said. "I want to use August to recuperate from the 3-Day."

David smiled. "You won't need a whole month," he said, chuckling. "It just feels like it right now."

"Still, I'll feel more comfortable with extra time."

When dinner was finished, Ross took out his micro recorder and his notebook and they started the interview. Emmy kept quiet at first as Ross went over David's background. Out of high school, he studied Business at San Francisco State, so he was local all the way.

"Emmy mentioned that you lost your wife to breast cancer," Ross said. It sounded intrusive, but it was probably just part of the job. "Do you have any children?"

Geez. I hadn't even thought of that.

David smiled. "Two. My daughter, Amanda, she's the oldest, lives in Sunnyvale. She works for Sun Microsystems. She's married and has a daughter, Jane. Yes, I'm a grandpa." He laughed. "My son Adam is a Junior at UC-Berkeley, in pre-med."

Emmy sat in shock. She just couldn't picture David as the father of adult children, let alone a grandfather!

"Congratulations," Ross said. He paused. "Your wife—was that how you got involved in the 3-Day?"

"Yes. Joanna." David stared down at the table. "We lost her in ninety-seven after a long fight."

He stopped, at a loss for words. Emmy was struck again at how much he'd loved his wife. And it was impossible not to see the similarities between Joanna Cook and Amelia Fleming. A great big lump formed in her throat and her fingers wrapped tightly around her garnet heart.

"It was... difficult to say the least. I don't know how she faced it with such peace, but... she was most beautiful at the very worst time. I think she tried to make it easier for the kids, I mean, it's impossible for children."

Ross cleared his throat.

"I know. I lost my dad to lung cancer."

David nodded. "I'm sorry."

"How did you hear about the 3-Day?"

"While she was sick, I heard about some of the American Cancer Society events and got involved in them. Someone sent me an email about the Avon Walk.

"At that time, there were no training walks at all in San Francisco. I'd been walking all over the City for years, so I put together some routes that met mileage demands and that was that. It was pretty bad at first. I was about thirty pounds overweight and I struggled to keep up with some of the people I was training, but I walked every day and by June I'd lost it all and built up muscle. Then we added speed."

Weight. That was something else they had in common.

The waitress stopped by and David ordered another beer and a shot of Bushmills whiskey. Ross and Emmy ordered mineral water.

It was a long interview. The pub filled with people and the noise level rose quite a bit, but Ross checked the recorder when he changed tapes and they could hear the questions and answers clearly, so they pressed on. After discussing a few specific routes, safety issues and techniques of walking, Ross finally arrived at the question Emmy most wanted answered.

"When I was in the 3-Day office," he said, "I was told that only a percentage of the funds raised actually goes to fight breast cancer. A substantial amount goes to Pallotta TeamWorks. I'm curious how you feel about that."

David smiled and shook his head. He looked up at the ceiling for a minute as if seeking divine help.

"Let me ask *you* a question," he said at last. "If a charity gives one hundred percent of their donations to a cause, how can they afford to pay their overhead costs?"

Ross thought about it. "I don't know."

David smiled. "All non-profits—like the Red Cross and the American Cancer Society—have to funnel a certain percentage of donations to cover overhead. Otherwise, how can they keep the organization running? It has to be paid for somehow. Emmy, you've been to the Cancer Society office?" She nodded. "How much do you think it costs? Let's start with personnel—the salaries."

She shook her head. "I don't know. A few hundred thousand. Probably more."

"What's the rent?"

"I don't know."

"It's enormous. And that's not even considering supplies, printing, office furniture, utilities, advertising, insurance. I'm an Office Manager. I can tell you that *everything* costs a lot. Where does the money come from?"

Emmy sat rapt, waiting to hear what was coming next. David paused for a moment, sipping his beer and staring at Ross over the foam.

"The American Cancer Society started their 'Making Strides' walks about five years ago and they have to enlist walkers from all over the United States just to raise three or four million dollars. Before Pallotta, there *was no* Breast Cancer 3-Day. They invented it. They got Avon to partner with them. I don't have the exact figures in front of me, but last year alone, they raised somewhere around fifty million dollars—*net*—they netted *fifty million dollars* to fight breast cancer. This year we're looking to top that total by another ten or twenty million."

He stopped to allow the figure to sink in.

"There are a lot of uninformed walkers out there who gripe about the amount of money that Pallotta makes by doing the walks, but Pallotta TeamWorks has brought in nearly ten times the amount of donations that were raised previously. I don't begrudge their income for one minute. They *earn* their fee."

He turned his head to Emmy with a bright stare. "Just wait till you see the level of support they provide. It'll knock you out. I think they coddle the walkers too much, but there are some walkers that need to be coddled. Some of them need it every step of the way. They may complain about Pallotta now, but believe me they'll be grateful for that first banana, for the free water, the sun screen and the port-o-potties, for a safe route, for breakfast, lunch and dinner—and a hot shower and a tent at the end of the day. They'll dance to the band that plays for them at night and have medics attend their blisters and masseuses rub their backs. Believe me, they'll be happy to have all of it."

He rubbed his jaw and looked around.

"Can you turn that thing off for a minute?"

Breaking out of his reverie, Ross reached over and turned the tape recorder off. David leaned forward and both of them leaned in to hear him.

"If some people have their way," he said quietly, "Avon's going to part ways with Pallotta and the whole thing's going to fall apart. Without Pallotta—without some company that has an actual stake in the success of the 3-Day—we'll never again raise as much money as we're raising now."

He leaned back in his chair and lifted his shot glass. After tilting it to Emmy and Ross in salute, he brought it to his lips and took the Bushmills in one gulp. Lowering the glass to the table, he thumped it against the linen.

"If you ask me," he said, "that's going to be a bloody shame."

27

Training Calendar of Team Aquatic Park

3-Day Simulation

6/29	Friday	23 Miles. 6 Hills.
6/30	Thursday	16 Miles. 4 Hills.
7/1	Sunday	20 Miles. 5 Hills.

Sunday, July 1

Sim—Day 3 *

She leaned her arms against the Cliff House sea wall, bent her left leg, and stretched her right leg out behind her. Muscles contracted all the way down to her Achilles tendon. Her thigh and calf bulged with

* See Map on Page 351.

the effort and she groaned. They were twelve miles into the twenty mile walk that capped the third and final day of the simulation.

Kat also put her hands on the wall, but she stretched both of her legs out behind her together and lowered herself until her stomach sagged way down toward the concrete patio. She held the position for a long time, then pushed herself up and blew out her breath.

"God, that felt good!" she said.

"What was that?" Emmy asked.

"My back, right down around the hips. It's been killing me for the last mile."

"Me, too. That works?"

Kat nodded. Reluctantly, Emmy lifted her left leg and placed it down by the right, then she leaned down and pushed her stomach closer to the patio concrete. She held the pose for at least ten seconds. As she pushed herself back up, relief flooded through her hips and lower back. Turning to Kat, she smiled.

"Neat trick."

A wave hit the rocks below and sent a splash of sea water over them, but neither moved. It felt good. After a short breather, they finished stretching, then trudged up the concrete stairs to the street. Each step sent a jolt of pain back up through her hips.

Those who were in their third consecutive day naturally gravitated together for support. Juliette looked completely wasted. Her skin was white and her normal exuberance was long gone. Kat hugged her and kissed her on the temple and Juliette managed a smile. Karen and Rhonda were haggard, but steady. Marianne looked like she had some energy, but on closer examination, Emmy saw her wince and knew she was hurting as much as the rest of them.

David had looked fine at the beginning, like it was any other day, but he had acquired a slight limp over the last few miles. In fact, she noticed that he had retrieved a runner's knee brace and now wore it over his right knee. She glanced at Kat and knew they were thinking the same thing: *Is he gonna walk home today after we finish?* Kat marched up to him and Emmy trailed behind her. When Kat spoke, her voice was low and menacing.

"I don't care what you say, David, I'm giving you a ride home today." He opened his mouth, but she raised her finger to his face. "Don't even try to argue with me!"

Kat turned and tromped past her. Emmy grinned. It was so funny to see little Kat badgering David that she actually laughed. He just shrugged and grinned at her.

"All I was gonna say was 'Thanks.'"

Up the street behind him, the second group approached. Janet led and they were making good time. Bertina was right behind her, head held high. She didn't even look at Emmy.

Ever since that damned donation, it's like I don't exist. She must know I made it and she's still pissed off.

Lauren, Alex and Darla were in the slow group and so was Rachel. She was the only other person to walk all three days. Emmy was really impressed that she'd toughed it out when she'd never trained with them before. David had already asked her to join the team, so she would finish her training with them.

It looked like they would all finish the twenty miles. They were well over half-way through and most of them didn't look half as worn out as Emmy felt.

Janet smiled as she walked up to them and hugged David. It was time for the changeover. Emmy wondered if she should volunteer to lead the second group. She'd never done it before, but it was past time she did. Everyone else had done it but her. She owed it to her teammates. When David looked around, she stepped forward.

"I'll do it," she said. Maybe it wasn't the best time to try, when she was burned out from three days of walking, but it felt right. Others had done it when they were tired, too.

"Are you sure?" David asked. "Next leg's all the way to California Pacific."

"I get ten extra minutes to rest while they take their break," she answered. To make her point, she smiled.

"You have your blister kit?"

"David, I have half the medical center in my backpack. Extra Gatorade. Extra food and water. I can do it."

He smiled at her. "Sure you can."

Janet turned off her cell phone, so Emmy fished hers out of the Whale and turned it on. She and David exchanged numbers while Janet stretched and hydrated, then the main group left for Golden Gate Park. It was an important moment for Emmy, watching them walk away. All this time, she had allowed others to lead the second group, while she got to walk up front with the team. Now, she was in charge of her own group for the first time ever.

I hope I can handle it.

Turning back, she looked around at the walkers and spotted Lauren, Alex, and Darla all stretching along the stairs. She was glad they were in her group. Truthfully, Lauren could probably lead them, but she had her own issues to deal with. She had walked the previous day and looked pretty worn out.

It gave a whole new meaning to Emmy's own exhaustion. Lauren had gone through enough with three different rounds of chemo and radiation, losing both breasts and fighting for her life and yet here she was, raising money and training to walk sixty miles.

Talk about giving back.

If Lauren could do all that, Emmy knew she could lead this group for five miles. She joined them and stretched again. After about ten minutes, she stood up and faced the group.

Moment of Truth.

"Alright, everybody," she called out, "Let's go."

She hoisted and secured the Whale to her back and led them down the sidewalk along Ocean Beach. Every step hurt now, but the break had revived her some. She kept a good pace. Lauren walked with her and they continued their conversation, but Emmy was hyper-aware of the time crunch and kept them moving smartly along.

Her plan was to pick up the pace in the park and see if the walkers responded. Surprisingly, almost everyone followed her lead. Walking faster also helped relieve the pain in her legs and hips, but it fatigued her even more. It felt like this weekend had been going on forever and it was never going to end.

She stumbled and Lauren quickly took her arm.

"You okay?" she asked.

"Sure," Emmy answered immediately. "Just a little tired."

Lauren smiled at her. "Three days kicks your butt, huh?" She nodded. "You're doing great," Lauren said. "The Walk will be a lot easier. It's really fun. There's a rush of adrenaline—so many people all walking for the same thing. It's great."

Her words made Emmy feel stronger and more awake. In four weeks she would be walking for real and it was exciting just to hear about it. It didn't take long for her to lead them into the Rose Garden for their break. She slung the Whale from her back, rummaged around, and pulled out her cell phone. Opening it up, she called David.

"Hey, Emmy!"

"Hey, David. We're at the Rose Garden."

"Damn, you've got 'em moving. We just left a few minutes ago. It's not far now to the medical center. You holding up?"

"Doing great," she lied. "We'll see you there soon."

She put her phone away and started to stretch. After a minute, she glanced up the path looking for her three stragglers. They were coming, but two of them were supporting the third. It was Rachel and the way she was limping, Emmy knew it was a blister. A shock of adrenaline rushed through her. She had never repaired a blister on her own, although she'd watched David do it a number of times now. It gave her shivers just thinking about slicing through one, but she was the leader and she had to handle the problem.

"Over here," she called out. They joined her and Rachel sat down in the grass. Emmy removed the shoe and looked at the sock. There was a large wrinkle across the ball of the foot.

"Wrinkle," she said, trying to sound like David. "From now on, make sure you pull your socks up after you stretch."

Rachel nodded, but Emmy saw the fright on her face: her eyes were full of tears just waiting to escape.

"It'll be okay," Emmy said. "We're gonna fix you up and you can walk back with the rest of us. Don't worry. It'll be fine."

Trying to keep her fingers from trembling, she opened the Whale and removed the blister kit. She pulled off the sock and took a long look at the nasty thing. It wasn't big, which was good, but Rachel had been walking on it for a while. There was a lot of fluid inside. Emmy put her supplies in order: a single-edged razor blade, gauze, moleskin, tape, and Neosporin.

"Lauren, would you to hold her foot?" Silently, Lauren moved into position and lifted Rachel's foot. "A little higher."

Emmy picked up the razor blade and took a deep breath.

Do it fast. Do it precisely. No wavering.

Looking squarely at the blister, she raised the blade, then, remembering David's advice, she glanced up at Rachel with a confident smile.

"You might want to grit your teeth. It's gonna hurt for a second."

Holding Rachel's heel in her left hand, she brought the blade up to the skin and swiftly cut straight down through the center of the blister.

"Ow!" Rachel jerked her foot and Emmy panicked for a moment. Had she cut too deep? She looked at the wound and didn't see any blood. "Oh," Rachel sighed, "God that feels good."

Emmy breathed out, too. *Thank goodness.* Smiling, she cut away the excess skin, slathered on Neosporin and prepared her moleskin. It just took a minute to dress the wound. She wound the tape around and around the foot, nice and snug.

"It's gonna hurt some," she said, "so take short steps. Try not to push off on it too hard." She gave the full lecture on care and Rachel's face was lit with a beautiful smile. She'd done a good job. *A damned good job!* Maybe her hands had trembled just a little, but not enough to draw blood. She put all of her supplies away, then drank deeply from her Gatorade bottle. After a few minutes of stretching, she checked her watch. It was already time to go.

"Alright everybody, let's move," she called out.

The group reassembled and she led them on through the park. Lauren moved up beside her again. Smiling, she reached over and patted Emmy on the shoulder.

"Handled like a pro," she said. "You should lead your own training walks."

Emmy blew out a breath as she took another painful step.

"Thanks," she answered. "I think I'll leave that to David."

They laughed and continued on through the park. At Stanyan Street, she looked behind them. Rachel moved resolutely with the others, not leaning on anyone.

Rachel Timmons will make it.

In spite of her protesting legs and swollen feet, Emmy kept the group walking at a good pace all the way to California Pacific. She felt a surge of pride when she brought them in. She had done her duty and done it well.

In the bathroom, she felt light-headed. Was she hydrating enough? She opened the Whale, pulled out a bottle of Gatorade and drank deeply. When she got back outside, she started to stretch.

"Okay, everybody," David said. "I'm taking Rachel on the easy route. Anyone who wants is welcome to join us."

It was tempting. Looking over at Kat, Emmy saw her thinking about it, too. Juliette sat on a bench, white and totally drained. Karen and Rhonda stood holding each other up. Marianne bent over and touched the sidewalk with her palms. She stood that way for a moment, then brought herself erect, staring off into the distance. Was it possible that she was considering the easy route? Marianne shook her arms, trying to get the numbness out of them. Abruptly, she slapped her palms together and turned to face the group, her mind made up.

"So," she said. "Anybody up for Pacific hill?"

Juliette pushed herself to her feet and hobbled slowly over to Marianne.

"I don't think I can do it," she said in a small, trembling voice.

Karen and Rhonda joined them, then Kat and Emmy. They wrapped their arms around each other, the six of them forming a huddle. Closing her eyes, Marianne blew out a long breath.

"We're almost home," she said. "Two and a half miles and it's over. Three days done. Three days. We'll only walk this far together one more time." She opened her eyes and looked around at them. "I've been in this building twice now, fighting an uphill battle against cancer. It makes the Pacific hill look like a puny pimple. You can do whatever you want and I don't care one way or another, but I'm gonna beat that fuckin' hill!"

Karen and Rhonda barked out weary chuckles and the rest of them joined in. Kat put her head next to Marianne's.

"*I'm* gonna beat it!"

"Me too," Emmy said, putting her head next to Kat's.

Karen leaned her head in. "Let's beat it!"

Rhonda looked up at them. She closed her eyes and rested her head next to her mother's.

"I'm in."

Juliette looked around at the five of them, her eyes moist. Then she put her head against the others to complete the circle.

"I love you guys," she said. Sucking in a breath that was half-sob, she raised her voice. "Let's beat that fuckin' hill!"

When the huddle broke, they turned and started up the street. It didn't matter that there wasn't a team around them—*they* were the team. They were six women who had walked hundreds of thousands of steps side by side. Now there was still one more hill.

They turned north on Spruce Street, pushed themselves up a short hill, then dropped down toward the Presidio, all the way down to Pacific Street. One by one, they turned up the alley and faced the little monster.

In silence, they moved forward.

Exhausted, her muscles aching with each step, Emmy pushed on. It wasn't difficult during the gentle slope at the beginning. She kept putting one foot in front of the other until the incline became a burden, then she slowed down. The six women were spread out on the hill, with Marianne leading and Kat right behind her. Karen and Rhonda were in front of Emmy and Juliette brought up the rear.

Emmy worked and worked. All she could think about was how good it would feel to stand on top of the damned thing. It would be the best thing ever.

Before the last big push, she had to stop at Presidio Avenue because a car was coming. She turned to look down behind her. Juliette had stopped about thirty paces back. At a respectable distance behind her, Tom led Team Aquatic Park. He halted the group and they all stood looking at Juliette.

Emmy focussed on her, too. She stood absolutely still, her hands on her hips, staring up at the hill with tears streaming down her face. It made Emmy think about the day when she had been so dehydrated and Juliette had dropped back to help her, staying with her, and making sure she made it.

It was gonna hurt, but she had to do it. Step by step, she lowered herself back down the hill. When she reached Juliette, she wrapped an arm around her and leaned her head close.

"You can do it," she whispered. "We'll do it together, okay?"

Juliette sniffled and nodded.

Taking the first step forward, they began to struggle up the hill together, holding each other tight. Step by step, they pushed and pushed. They stopped to rest at Pacific Avenue. Tom didn't allow anyone on the team to pass them. He was honoring them by allowing them to beat the hill together. Finally, when they were within twenty paces of the top, Emmy heard someone clapping. Then more hands joined together and there was cheering. David's group had joined the others and they were all cheering.

Emmy and Juliette took the final few steps to the top of the hill and were encircled in the arms of Marianne, Kat, Karen and Rhonda.

Juliette sobbed and they all held her.

It was a stunning moment. Emmy knew with complete certainty that they would be friends for life—all six of them—and they would always be there for each other.

It was the strongest bond she had ever felt in her life and she never wanted to let it go.

Ever.

28

Training Calendar of Team Aquatic Park

7/15	Sunday	13 Mile Hill Walk.
7/21	Saturday	8 Mile Hill Walk.
7/22	Sunday	7 Mile Flat Walk.

Tuesday, July 24

"So." Barb raised her head and smiled. "You're ready?"

"As ready as I'll ever be. Except for packing. I'm gonna do that Thursday morning before Kat picks me up."

"When is she coming for you?"

"Ten o'clock."

"Well, that should give you plenty of time. Assuming you don't oversleep."

Emmy chuckled. "I'll be lucky if I sleep at all!"

"I'm very proud of you," Barb said. Her smile was genuine. It seemed weird, but Emmy had actually gotten to like her. She had immensely changed Emmy's life with the 3-Day. And, now, it seemed like she really cared.

"Thanks."

"You brought your shirt, like I asked?"

"Yes," Emmy answered, reaching into her bag. *Abstract. Always in the abstract.* She unfolded the shirt and passed it over. Barb closely examined the signatures. At the bake sale, Emmy had added her mother and sisters' signatures and even got her dad to sign it. From work, there were the signatures of Tina, Joanna, Marcy, and even Jack Markham. There was hardly any space, but Emmy handed over the Sharpie. Barb's eyes were a little moist.

"I'm not sure I belong in this group," she said.

Emmy smiled. "Oh, you belong."

Barb located a small free space and wrote her name. After a minute, she turned it over. Her eyes grew round as she looked at the photo of Amy. It made an impact.

"She was a stunning woman," Barb said. "An inspiration. When are you going to wear it?"

"Day Two."

"What a shame I won't be able to see it on you."

"I'd wear it Sunday, but we're all wearing our team shirts. I'll get a photo for you."

Emmy's fingers trembled, just a little, but Barb saw it.

"I've been thinking," she said, holding the shirt in her lap, "about a conversation we had once about forgiveness."

I remember. It really pissed me off.

"Yes, you were wondering if I'd ever forgiven Mom. Well, I have. We've really made peace now and it's good."

"When did that happen?"

"At the bake sale. I think she's changed. Or I've changed."

"Perhaps a little of both."

"Maybe..."

They sat quietly for a moment, then Barb raised her head.

"Well, that leaves one person left for you to forgive."

Emmy tingled. *Geez. Dad, Dean, Mom. Who else is there?* She felt completely lost. It was a trap. She knew it, yet she couldn't stop herself from asking:

"Who?"

Barb lifted the shirt so the picture of Amy was facing her. It took a moment for her to figure it out, then her mouth gaped in astonishment.

"Why on earth would I have to forgive Amy?"

"I think you know why," Barb answered. *Like it's a sacred mystery*

I should already know. Emmy fumed. It was completely out of line. All the good grace she'd mustered for Barb was gone and she barely controlled her anger when she answered.

"God, I hate it when you do that! *Why*?"

Barb straightened up and looked Emmy square in the eyes.

"Because she left you when you needed her most."

"That's not fair! It's not like she had a choice."

"I'm not saying she did. I'm just saying she left you."

Emmy grabbed her carryall and snatched the shirt away. She turned toward the door, calling out over her shoulder as she left:

"Have you ever considered getting therapy?"

29

Day Zero

Thursday, July 26, 6:10 am

I guess it was inevitable.

Finally, after what seemed a lifetime, I dreamed about Amy again. My lost memory. It's frustrating that I can't get it over with and done. It's also scary because I don't really want to know how it ends. I don't want to know what happened.

I'd always been stopped right on the stairs of California Pacific. Then I made it past Grace, through the doors and into the building. Into the elevator. Into her room.

Last night, I remembered more. I stood near the door. Amy was in her bed, looking directly at me. I couldn't run. I couldn't breathe.

"There's nothing more to do," she said. "I'm going home."

It was overwhelming, I remember that now. I couldn't even think. I just stood, petrified with fear. I was going to lose her. Intense pain. Fear. Throbbing. I didn't hear anything she said after that until suddenly it was silent.

She said it would be the last time we saw each other.

I blacked out and then I woke up.

It's a shitty way to start Day Zero, but there you have it.

Now that I'm awake, I've got to shower and pack my new duffel bag. My fanny packs were named the Minnow and the Blowfish and my backpack has been the Whale. I couldn't think of anything bigger than a whale, so I named my duffel bag the Behemoth—and I have to get it packed before Kat and her dad get here at 10.

Big day. Here. Now.

It's time to start Day Zero.

30

Emmy bounced on her toes with her stomach tied in knots. She stood on the sidewalk in front of her apartment building next to the bulging Behemoth .

Three days. Sixty miles. Geez.

Day Zero. Registration. No turning back.

She checked her watch. Kat and her father should be arriving at any moment to take them to Santa Clara. Exhausted, yet excited.

Weird combination.

It had been a long morning, the highlight of which had been her weigh-in. Regardless of what might happen over the weekend, she'd topped out: twenty-six pounds lost and gone forever. Of course, it wasn't about weight. It was about checking in, whether it was walking or helping others or even therapy. It was about showing up.

Reaching down, she patted the blue and white Behemoth. There were two padded straps on one side, so she could carry it like the Whale, and also a single long strap so she could sling it over her shoulder. Kat had an identical bag that was pink and white. They'd bought them together in Chinatown during a lunch hour.

Packing it had been a second nightmare that had gobbled up her entire morning. It contained her air mattress and sleeping bag, her spare shoes, walking clothes for three days, the skirt and blouse she planned on wearing to the team dinner later that evening, as well as extra clean clothes for camp, and a mess of extra stuff, from underwear to make up.

The first effort at packing had ended with a loaded Behemoth and half of her stuff still spread out on the bed. She'd had to unpack, rethink the process, edit, and repack—and somehow she'd made it fit.

She patted the purse hanging from her shoulder. It also bulged, but with her cell phone, camera, and extra film, and all of her registration material. In her anxiety, she'd almost locked it in the apartment.

A blue Honda Civic with a white-haired Chinese man behind the wheel pulled up and double parked in front of the building. Kat jumped out of the passenger side as the trunk popped open.

"Hey, girl!" Kat grinned.

"Hi, Kat."

Emmy wrestled the Behemoth into the trunk next to Kat's. After a brief introduction to Kat's father, she settled into the back seat, while Kat climbed into the shotgun so she could give directions to Marianne's place.

As they passed through Golden Gate Park, Emmy remembered the day that Tina had signed her up. She hadn't thought she could ever walk sixty miles—and now, after seven months of training, she was actually going to do it. According to her training journal, when the next three days were over, she would top one thousand miles.

Geez! A thousand miles!

They picked up Marianne and headed for Santa Clara.

It was a fast drive down the peninsula on I-280. The freeway wound along the lee side of the ridgeline. Emmy took in the whole panorama, from way down at the Bay all the way up to the very top. It would be an ugly climb, that was for sure. She could make it, though. After all, she *had* to do it. In a way, she was eager for it.

The first day should be the worst—twenty-three and a half miles of flat heat, hedged in among twenty-five hundred people, but Hell Hill would be the real test. Of course, Day Three wouldn't be a picnic either. She felt amazed that she was actually doing this, but it was what she'd trained for and she definitely felt prepared.

The further south they drove, the more it seemed like a very, very long distance. They rolled through town after town: Daly City, San Bruno, Burlingame, San Mateo, Belmont, Redwood City, Palo Alto, Mountain View, and Sunnyvale, before entering Santa Clara.

It was a beautiful city, just north of San Jose, green and immaculate—even the streets looked brand new. Mr. Chen pulled the car into a long, U-shaped driveway at the Convention Center, came to a stop in a line of cars, and popped open the trunk. They jumped out to get their luggage. Mr. Chen came around to help.

"Thanks, Dad." Kat kissed him. "I love you!"

Famous last words.

Marianne and Emmy thanked him for the ride, then they joined the swarm of bodies moving into the complex and got in line to check in. A constant babble of conversation echoed through the large room, punctuated by shrill hoots and laughter. Most of the walkers were women, but there were plenty of men, too. And a lot of middle-aged and older people. Ross had asked her to document the event, so she took a lot of photos.

Separated from her friends by Walker Number assignments, Emmy found herself in a short line. In mere moments, she moved up to the desk to present her papers. The lady checking in gave her a dark blue lanyard with her laminated Walker card. It had the 3-Day logo and her Walker Number, 1110, in large, bold letters. As she draped it around her neck, she felt goosebumps rise on her arms. Her pink vinyl bracelet was locked onto her wrist, then she signed the final Waiver of Liability and received her checklist. This was it. She couldn't turn and run any more. She had to do it.

When the three were reunited, they signed up for the first open slot to watch the safety video, but it was still over an hour away so they went to get tent assignments and luggage tags. Kat and Emmy were assigned Row A, Number 3.

"Hey!" Kat cried. "Good luck! Right up front!"

"What difference does it make?" Emmy asked, looping her luggage tag around a strap on the Behemoth.

Kat giggled. "It really comes in handy if you have to pee in the middle of the night." It was noon already, so they followed others through the mess line to a little park and settled down in a grassy area to eat. The warm afternoon and buzzing of conversation combined to make her feel lazy.

After the safety video, she was dead tired, but went on to tent instruction. Even though Kat said she knew how to put the tent together, Emmy wanted to pull her own weight, so she watched the instructor closely, then got down on her knees to practice laying it out, assembling the poles and threading them through the support flaps.

Through it all, she kept taking photos—not just for Ross, but for future years when she would be able to look at the pictures and remember everything.

Finally, it was time to check in at the hotel. Gathering their luggage, they joined the throng of people moving back and forth between the Convention Center and hotel.

The hotel, much like the city, was beautiful. When they arrived on the third floor, Marianne headed down the hall to the room she shared with Janet. Kat keyed them into their own room, then stopped, temporarily stunned at the luxury. She dropped her duffel, sprinted across the room, and threw herself on the bed by the window.

"I could live here," she cried through laughter.

"I don't think we could afford this," Emmy answered, looking in the bathroom.

The phone rang and Kat picked it up. Everyone was down in the bar and David wanted them to stop by once they were settled. Unpacking was simple—just the few things they would need overnight. Emmy hung her skirt and blouse; she'd need to iron them before dinner. Dividing the bathroom sink, they each claimed a half and were soon ready to leave.

When the elevator opened at the lobby, they heard the cacophony of a hundred conversations coming from the bar down the hall. A large, open area, it was fully packed with walkers unwinding from registration.

A loud guffaw from the back revealed the location of Tom O'Laughlin, so they followed it and found the team gathered around four tables in the far corner. Plates of appetizers were spaced across the tables, along with pints of beer, mixed drinks, and a few sodas.

"Welcome!" David called out over the chaos.

"Hey!" Tom cried. "Grab a seat."

The only visible waitress was completely overwhelmed, so they pulled up chairs to wait. Five or six conversations were going at once and it was difficult to follow any of them. David sat with his back to a window on a long padded bench, with Janet next to him on one side and Tom on the other with Michael.

Surprisingly, the waitress swooped in and took their order right away. Tom leaned in close to Michael and several other heads inclined that way, so Emmy scooted closer. Tom grinned at Michael, his eyes twinkling.

"So tell me," he asked casually, "why are gynecologists never unemployed?"

"Gynecologists are never unemployed?" Michael asked.

"Never," Tom replied, grinning.

Michael smiled and gave it some thought, but looked lost. Emmy couldn't think of anything either. "I give up," Michael answered. "Why are gynecologists never unemployed?"

"Because wherever you go," Tom said, "there's always an opening."

"Whoa!" Michael sputtered, cracking up. Emmy laughed with them, but she understood now why Kat had warned her against Tom's gynecological jokes.

Kat moved over to join Karen, Rhonda, and some others, so Emmy followed. Karen had heard rumors the route was changed from the last year, so there was rampant speculation. Looking around, Emmy saw familiar faces. Joy, Ellen, Juliette and Rachel were there, but someone was missing.

Emmy scooted closer to David. "Where's Bertina?"

He drank from his beer, then leaned in close to her.

"She'll be here tomorrow," he said.

"Not tonight?"

"Nope. Can't afford it."

"She should be here." It pissed her off. They should have done something so she could make the team dinner. Taken up a collection or something. She leaned in to David.

"It's not right," she said. "She should be here with us."

"Listen," he replied, leaning close to her. "Tom offered to pay for the hotel and the dinner, but she refused. Said she wasn't going to take charity." He leaned back. "I know where she's coming from." He tilted his beer to her. "I respect it."

"It's still not right," Emmy repeated.

A silence stretched out between them, much like the silence between Emmy and Bertina since the anonymous donation. *She must know I did it. I bet she hasn't forgiven me.* Somehow, it enflamed her anger. She had done a good thing and yet Bertina was still punishing her for it.

She finished her beer. All the good feeling was gone and she was just dead tired. She turned to Kat.

"I need to get some rest before dinner."

"Yeah, me, too."

Upstairs, Kat turned on the TV, stretched out on her bed, and started flipping through channels. Emmy dug out the iron and board to press her skirt and blouse. When she was finished, she peeled off her jeans and pulled back the covers on her bed.

"If I fall asleep, would you wake me up at five-thirty?"

"Sure," Kat answered.

She climbed between the sheets and closed her eyes.

31

"Hey! Wake up, Emmy! It's five-thirty!"

Kat shook her. *Geez, I just laid down.*

"Okay, okay!" she answered. Her mind was foggy and she felt numb. Her tongue was dry. Sitting up in bed, she rubbed her eyes.

"Man, you snore like a horse," Kat said.

"I don't snore."

"Girl, you snore like one of them vacuum pumps."

Emmy laughed. "Hey, I'm tired. Give me a break." She pulled off the covers, got out of bed, and headed for the bathroom.

"I'll lay you ten to one Ross wears ear plugs!"

Washing her face woke her up a little, but she was still blurry as she dressed, brushed her hair, and put on some light make-up. She stepped in front of the full-length mirror. Kat watched from her seat on the bed.

"How do I look?" Emmy asked.

"You look great!" Kat smiled. "I knew you were losing weight, but I had no idea how much."

"Thanks!"

Kat stood, her sleek, long black hair falling over her shoulders. In her shiny, red satin dress, she was beautiful.

"You look amazing," Emmy said.

They stood side by side at the mirror.

"We clean up pretty good," Kat replied, squeezing her shoulder.

The hallway was alive with noise. Several doors were wedged open and music blasted up and down the corridor, punctuated with laughter and chatter. It was a party.

The restaurant was certainly elegant.

"I'm glad we dressed up," Kat whispered.

Two large tables had been pushed together and the team was spread out around them. Kat and Emmy took two seats near David.

"I'm recommending red wine and pasta," he said.

Tom leaned over. "The red wine is medicinal."

Karen laughed. "Yeah, right!"

"It is!" Janet cried. "It's full of antioxidants. Good for the heart!"

"And the pasta?" Emmy asked.

"Body loves carbs before a big workout," David answered. "Turns directly to glucose. Instant fuel."

In her tradition of always following David's advice, Emmy went with red wine and ravioli, a popular choice around the table. She ordered a side salad, too. *Gotta get some veggies.*

Karen looked at David. "You hear about the route changes?"

"Yeah, it'll be convoluted at first. And be prepared to ride the train partway."

"No way!" Kat cried.

"It's still sixty miles."

The tables erupted in chatter. No one was happy with the idea, but it didn't take long for the conversation to move on. Everyone was too pumped up to let it bring them down.

"As long as they have biscuits and gravy for breakfast, I'm okay," Tom said. "Man, but that was so good last year!"

After dinner, they talked for a long while until Janet stood, facing them. "I'd like to make a toast," she said.

"Hear! Hear!" Tom seconded.

The room grew quiet and Janet lifted her glass.

"For everything he's given us—for the second year in a row—I toast our fearless leader, with the wickedest hill walks in the city of San Francisco!" She waited for the applause to die down. "To David Cook!" He reached out and clinked her glass, then there was clinking around the table and sipping of wine in contentment. As Janet sat back down, Tom stood and raised his glass.

"I'd like to make a toast, too."

Emmy looked up at him, expecting a joke, but his face was serious and thoughtful, as it had been on that day when he had told her about Jessica Timmons.

"About a month ago," he continued, "I saw one of the most incredible things I've ever seen in my life. Six dedicated women pulled themselves up the Pacific Street hill at the end of nearly sixty miles of walking." The room was silent and all eyes were on Tom. "Women never get the credit they deserve for courage and perseverance. Well, those six women showed a hell of a lot of courage.

"Here's to them: Marianne, Kat, Karen, Rhonda, Emmy, and Juliette!"

Emmy sat in silence as glasses clinked. His words had meant so much to her. And now, suddenly, she felt sad. The evening was almost over and she didn't want it to end. She didn't want any of it to end.

When the noise settled down, David rose and lifted his brandy glass. Everyone fell quiet as his gaze ranged around the room, taking in each person.

"I just want to say thanks to everybody. You've shown a lot of dedication, week in and week out, dragging yourselves down to the park, up and down hills, across the City and back, getting ready for this thing. It takes a special person to make that kind of commitment."

A rosy quiet settled over the team. People glanced at each other, smiling, and heads nodded. David cleared his throat.

"I also commend you for the job you've done raising money to fight breast cancer. You've all raised a hell of a lot for the cause and, personally, I thank you very, very much."

As he paused, a gleam came into his eyes.

"Now, a final bit of advice, while I have a captive audience." He grinned. "Word has it we might reach three thousand walkers this year." There was a rush of excited chatter and David waited for it to ebb. He cleared his throat again.

"When you get out on the streets tomorrow, be sure to respect everyone. Respect the crew members, who donate their valuable time, the police who protect us, and the public who come to cheer us on. It's special for everyone.

"And although we've trained to walk fast, take some time over the next three days to enjoy this thing. It's a wonderful, amazing event, the 3-Day." Emmy's throat tightened and her eyes grew moist. "It may not be around forever. Take it all in, savor it. It's precious. Never forget that."

He was silent for a moment.

"So, for the final toast of the evening, I'd like you all to rise and join me."

One by one, they each stood and raised their glasses to David. He lifted his brandy glass and looked around the room. A smile lifted the corners of his mouth and his eyes twinkled behind the wire-rimmed glasses.

"To the end of breast cancer!"

Their voices rose as one:

"To the end of breast cancer!"

32

Day One

Friday, July 27

Kat and Emmy stepped out into a cool, sunny morning and joined the massive flow of bodies swarming toward the Convention Center.

Weaving their way through three thousand people was no easy feat, but it felt familiar. *Clever David: Bay to Breakers. It was prep.* They found the luggage trucks and checked in their duffel bags, then headed for the meeting spot. They passed a tent with volunteers passing out bananas and granola, so they took some and a couple of bottles of water, then headed to the meeting area.

The team had voted to see the ceremony, rather than meeting at the starting line, so they gathered inside the center, as close to a side door as possible. Hopefully, they wouldn't have to start in the middle of the crowd; already, the plaza outside was full of walkers massing around the starting line.

Juliette stood on Emmy's right and Kat and Marianne were on her left, with Rachel further down the line. Joy and Ellen, Michael, Bertina and Lauren, with Alex and Darla, stood behind her. Janet, Karen, and Rhonda were in front of her and David and Tom waited by the door. She glanced at Bertina, but her nod of greeting wasn't acknowledged.

It was hard to wait. A chant started. Walkers on her left called out "Three!" and it was answered on her right with "Day!" It got louder and everyone clapped rhythmically with the echoing calls.

"Three!"

"Day!"

"Three!"

"Day!"

"Three!"

"Day!"

Emmy shivered, tingling all over. She jumped up and down from sheer excitement. The lights dimmed and music blared from massive speakers. She caught flashes of a man in a red shirt walking on one of the elevated walkways, carrying a flag. He said something, but his microphone was muffled.

A woman from the Avon Breast Cancer Crusade stepped up to the lectern. She welcomed them to the 3-Day and announced that the preliminary numbers for fundraising showed that the San Francisco Walk had already raised *five-point-five million dollars* to fight breast cancer.

A great cry erupted in the room and Emmy screamed with everyone else. Regardless of how much the Pallotta fee might be, they had raised an enormous amount of money.

Next, a small group of breast cancer survivors walked along one of the elevated walkways. They held hands forming a circle, the center representing the spirits of breast cancer victims, the spirits of those who had lost their lives: "mothers, daughters, sisters, aunts..." Emmy looked around. That was mostly everyone, including her, but she couldn't allow herself to get caught up in memory.

I won't.

The final speech was inspiring and it built to an ending in which the speaker hammered on the goal: to end breast cancer forever. Emmy felt tight all over and fought to overcome it. She heard sniffling all around. Juliette wiped her eyes. Behind them, Lauren stood erect, her eyes gleaming.

We've got to start walking or I'll go nuts. Let's go!

"And now, my friends," the speaker cried, "the San Francisco Avon Breast Cancer 3-Day officially begins!"

As his words echoed through the room, David and Tom pushed quickly through the door. Emmy turned to follow, but there was already a bottleneck of bodies. She and Juliette were not far behind the guys, but as people pressed against them, the team became separated. Emmy stayed close to Juliette, but it was slow going. As they emerged into the sun, she slipped her sunglasses down from her baseball cap. Bodies were pressed tightly together and funneled slowly from the large plaza toward the starting line. All around, there was the white noise of chatter, cheering, hooting, and shouting. There was a mob of supporters around the starting line cheering them on. It was total chaos.

There was nothing to do but let it work itself out. Juliette took her hand and they moved forward slowly. Swiveling her head, Emmy saw Kat, Marianne, Janet, and Michael all further back, moving forward at a snail's pace. As the two girls approached the starting line, it became a little less crowded, then they surged under the arch and moved forward into the actual 3-Day Walk. She peered up ahead of them, but there was no sign of David or Tom.

It's time to make hay.

She and Juliette exchanged glances and picked up their pace, but were abruptly stopped in a line of people waiting for a red light. It took two changes of the light before they even got up to the curb. They waited, then moved forward, then were stopped by another red light. And another. Just as David had said, it was very frustrating. Emmy held her camera in the air and took photos of the lines.

Finally, they emerged into a park where they could finally stretch it out. For a long time, their calls echoed back and forth:

"On your right!"

"On your left!"

They shot past other walkers, but the park ended way too soon. There was no sign of David or Tom and now she couldn't even see teammates behind them. Entire blocks full of walkers were stranded between stoplights.

There was a flash of blue as a large Hispanic officer with the San Jose Police pedaled up on his bicycle and stopped traffic. Another officer across the street did the same so the logjam of bodies could clear up. Somebody blew a shrill wolf whistle and the officer laughed.

"Thanks!" Emmy called out as they shot across the street. He smiled and waved, then the cars began to honk. At first, she thought they were upset with the traffic, but then there was a shout:

"Go Walkers!"

They weren't angry. They were honking *in support!*

She waved at the cars and continued on at the best pace she could muster. Block after block, it was stop and wait, then charge forward, then stop and wait again. The Police swooped in and they surged forward. It was a massive effort. At last, they were ushered into a park by cheering crew members, holding out bottles of water and Gatorade. There was a sign that read, "Grab 'N Go," so they each grabbed a bottle of water in one hand and Gatorade in the other, and went.

They were into a residential neighborhood now and it was much easier going, even with all the bodies taking up the sidewalks. They picked up speed and barreled along. It was exhilarating to stride out. Soon, Emmy was coated in sweat and it felt great.

The miles added up and they came to the first Pit Stop. It was in a little park and manned by volunteers dressed in grass skirts, shouting encouragement. There were bins of iced bottles of water and Gatorade and bowls of bananas, apples, and yogurt. A line of port-o-potties stood along a fence. Emmy had finished about half of her water and Gatorade, so she mixed them and tossed the empty into a recycle bin.

"David!" It was Juliette.

Emmy turned to see her running toward a tree where David and Tom stood stretching. The four of them hugged like they hadn't seen each other in years. Tom's laughter rang through the park.

"Now we're getting to the good stuff," David said.

"Where are we?"

"I think we're in Mountain View or Los Altos," Tom answered.

"We gotta go," David said. "Catch you at the next break."

As they strode off, the girls began to stretch—they didn't want to get too far behind. Emmy's legs had finally stiffened and she knew they had gone about seven miles. The sun blasted away at them, so they put on more sunscreen. Before they left, Kat and Marianne arrived. The four hugged and quickly exchanged information before the arrivals started to stretch.

Setting off up the street, Emmy and Juliette made excellent time. There were a few mild inclines, but no hills. They continued to pass walkers, but it was no longer the huge crowd they'd faced at the beginning. Emmy finished her Gatorade cocktail and picked up replacements at the next Grab 'N Go.

Without the Whale—only the Minnow now—she flew along the street. There weren't many stoplights and by constantly looking ahead and to the side, they timed entering intersections and moved through them quickly. They had gone all directions throughout the morning, but she saw that they were now definitely going northwest.

We're heading for San Francisco!

The public cheering dropped off, but there were still a few places where it picked back up. Sometime during the blur of miles, they passed a truck blaring out the song "Pretty Woman" on a tape loop.

The bicycle cops showed up, disappeared, reappeared at larger intersections and it really helped with their speed.

They tagged up with David and Tom at the next Pit Stop, then with Kat and Marianne before they left. The distance was getting shorter between all of them and they were hopeful that soon they would all be walking together. During the next leg of the walk, it became increasingly apparent that they were somewhere up around Palo Alto. Eventually, Kat and Marianne caught up with them.

"You guys must be really humping it!" Emmy said.

"Got caught at lights," Kat gasped.

"Had to make up ground." Marianne was panting, too.

"We hit all the lights, too," Juliette said. She smiled. "Guess we're not 'humping' it like you two."

As they approached the break area, all four of them were laughing. David and Tom were waiting for them and Emmy started to relax. They were finally a team again.

"Some of the others aren't far behind us," Marianne said. "At least nine or ten of us should team up after lunch."

"I wonder where lunch is at?" Juliette asked.

One of the Crew raised her head.

"It's your next stop."

"Already?" Emmy asked. She checked her wrist watch. It wasn't even eleven o'clock yet. "We're making great time."

After stretching, the six of them headed out together. Kat fell into step beside Emmy and glanced over with a smile.

"I missed you," she said. "It just isn't the same without you on my left."

"Me, too." Emmy grinned. Things were back to normal.

Within thirty minutes, they walked into the lunch area. It was set up in a little plaza in the middle of a large park. Large white tents, open on the sides, dotted the area. Some of them served lunch, some were medical aid tents and an area for massage.

At last, Emmy had to urinate, so she made her way with some trepidation toward the line of port-o-potties set up against a fence. It was her first trip inside one and she wasn't sure what to expect. She opened the door and stepped into a small space. It was green and the thin walls allowed the sunlight to filter in. It was very sanitary and although the chemical smell wasn't exactly rosy, at least it didn't stink.

She picked up lunch—a small sandwich, a bag of chips, apple sauce, and a cookie—and joined the team at a table. No one spent any time savoring the food, but the conversation was lively. Marianne estimated that they should make camp by three-thirty, which would leave them lots of time to set up for the evening.

As they ate, Janet, Michael, Joy and Ellen arrived. The four of them quickly ate, stretched, and hydrated, then the eight members of the team set off briskly together.

Now, the walking was fun. David set the pace at four miles an hour and they flew along the streets and sidewalks. Houses, businesses, endless intersections—it was a complete blur. They didn't pass many other walkers—it meant they were getting up toward the front and that meant early camp.

When they stretched at the next Pit Stop, Emmy definitely felt the mileage. It was strange that it had taken so long for her muscles to hurt. It had been a full month since the sim and she actually felt much better than during a normal training walk.

"I'm not hurting as much as usual," she remarked.

"Me, neither," Kat replied, grinning. "No hills."

Emmy stared at her. "That's right. Hadn't thought of that."

"What'd I tell you the first day you walked up into the bleachers?" Kat's grin was infectious.

"An easy 3-Day!" Emmy grinned back.

They slapped a high five and set off again.

As the day wore on and the miles piled up, she hurt more and more.

Maybe "easy" had been overstating the case. Her hip joints were swollen and her feet ached, but every time they stopped to stretch, her muscles responded. And when they set off again she felt good and loose.

Shortly before two o'clock, they approached a Caltrain station. A crew member pointed them up onto the platform and they walked past a large sign that read, "Menlo Park." There were five other walkers waiting on the platform.

"It's true," Janet said. "They're putting us on a train."

"At least we know we're at Menlo Park," Marianne replied.

David walked on down ahead of Tom, who raised his hand. "Pardon me, boy," he said. "Is this the Transylvania Station?"

Stopping in his tracks, David turned back. "Ya, ya," he replied, using an accent, "Track 29. Can I give you a shine?"

Tom laughed. "Quick on the uptake, my friend."

Janet groaned. "Oh, no. Geez. Here comes *Young Frankenstein*."

Looking down the tracks, Emmy saw the train approaching. Michael strolled over to Tom and glanced back at us.

"Igor," he said, "help me with the bags."

"Certainly," Tom answered, doing Groucho Marx. "You take the blond, I'll take the one with the turban."

The guys laughed raucously, but only Marianne joined in. Emmy had seen the movie—and it was funny—but she just didn't find it as hilarious as the guys. The seating on the train was comfortable, so everybody kicked back, slouching and draping themselves across the seats. Michael actually put his feet up in the window.

"Geez," Tom quipped, "if I'd known they were gonna send us first class, I'd never have trained with you guys."

"Beats the Pacific hill," Ellen remarked.

Tom glanced up at her. "I thought you loved the Pacific hill?"

"Yeah, love it to death," she replied. Tom grinned.

"You'll get your hill," David said. "Don't worry."

Emmy realized that she hadn't taken any photos in a while, so she broke out her camera and took pictures of everyone. They posed for group shots, then others brought out cameras and everybody got a group pose.

The train rolled into the San Carlos station and they quickly scrambled off. Day One had been so much better than the simulation that Emmy wondered if David had deliberately made the sim harder. *But who cares?* The result was that the actual thing seemed pretty easy.

At last, they hit a long stretch along El Camino Real and kicked it up into the next gear. Emmy checked her watch. It was almost two thirty. They were in south San Mateo, not that far from camp. She yearned to wash off the accumulated sweat and grit and sunscreen, to set up their tent, pump up the air mattress, and relax.

She heard clapping and cheering up ahead and checked her watch again. It was three-fifteen. They were walking up a long drive through a funnel of crew members slapping their hands. There was a gate across the road, with a sign that read, "Bay Meadows."

It was the horseracing stadium—camp!

Twenty-three miles and we finished in less than eight hours!

33

Everyone around her was whooping and yelling, so Emmy cried out, too, slapping the crew's hands as they passed through the gate.

The luggage trucks were close by, so after their warm-down, Emmy and Kat retrieved their duffels, picked up a tent, and joined the others, following signs that led around the grandstand, down into a long tunnel, and up a ramp onto the grassy infield. It was laid out in a huge grid and right up front was Row A. They were in the third space over. Less than twenty tents had been set up. David and Tom were next to Marianne and Janet. They were pretty close to Emmy and Kat, but Joy and Ellen were clear across the field and Michael was in the next area code.

Their tent set-up was lightning fast. Kat spread out the tent while Emmy assembled the poles. They threaded them through the supports and twisted the entire tent upright. Kat balanced and anchored it while Emmy assembled the rain fly. In moments, they were done. It looked good and felt sturdy.

Every time she had to bend over or squat, it hurt, but the aerobic activity was good for her and she knew it. They took turns using the foot pump to inflate their air mattresses, placing them on opposite sides of the tent, then unrolled their sleeping bags.

Kat threw herself down on her bed and sighed.

"Wonderful!"

Leaning down, Emmy fell onto her air mattress. It was so soft. *God, but it feels good!* Sleeping would not be a problem, provided Tom didn't keep them awake all night. Kat dug out her toiletry bag and a towel, so Emmy followed suit. Grabbing a change of clothes, they flung their towels over their shoulders and set off up the tunnel.

The others joined them trudging back to the huge main camp: a series of large, white tents open to the air. Crew members were still assembling the gigantic dining tent, putting up long rows of tables and folding chairs. It would hold hundreds of people. There were medical tents, massage areas, a store, and several others that Emmy couldn't immediately identify.

The showers were inside large truck trailers. The generators that ran them were loud enough to be a nuisance, but she gladly put up with it to have a hot shower. It was easy to languish a bit, but others were waiting, so she put on shorts and a tee shirt and they headed back to the tents.

"What do we do till dinner?" Emmy asked.

Joy turned to her. "We're going up front to cheer the walkers into camp."

"I'm gonna look for lost souls," Kat answered, "and help them set up their tents. You'd be surprised how many lost souls there truly are."

David and Tom were already helping others, so Emmy and Kat stored their gear, then got to work. Rachel, Karen and Rhonda finally made it into camp.

Behind them, she saw Bertina, carrying a suitcase and dragging a tent bag. Although she was already working with two women, Emmy kept her eye on Bertina, who was wandering around toward a section at the back. *At least she made it into camp before her tentmate.*

Emmy finished up, then turned to see Bertina open her tent bag and dump the contents on the ground. *Well,* she thought, *if she's still mad at me, I can't make it any worse.* Marching back to join her frenemy, Emmy squat and spread out the main tent. Bertina grabbed it away and straightened it out, so Emmy took the poles and began assembling them.

Bertina stopped, with a look fit to melt plastic. It pierced and it hurt and it pissed Emmy off, but she kept working. After a moment, Bertina stooped down and they worked together in silence, threading the poles, twisting the tent upright and completing the rain fly. When it was done, they stood back to look at it.

"Looks good," Emmy said. "Tough. It'll hold up."

"Thanks," Bertina remarked grudgingly.

"Just pass it on," Emmy answered. "Help someone else. That's how it works."

They stared at each other.

"Is that so?"

"Yeah," Emmy answered. "I'm sorry if I pissed you off. I'm sorry if helping you out was a capital crime, but lots of people helped me out and I never got pissed at them. You're here, that's what's most important. You're here. Pass it on."

She ran out of breath and went silent.

The corners of Bertina's mouth twitched with humor and her brown eyes twinkled. "So it wasn't Mayor Willie," she said. "I knew you'd crack. You shouldn't ever try to keep a secret, girl. You're no good at it." She grinned. "I'll pass it on. After I shower."

Kat called to her across the field.

"Hey, Emmy! It's nearly five-thirty. Wanna go up front?"

They trudged back through the tunnel and joined the crowd cheering the last of the walkers. It was a lot more fun than Emmy had thought it would be. It felt good to give the walkers at the tail end a boost. They had been on the trail for ten hours. Most of them were hurting and they looked exhausted, limping along, assisted by friends. Some who had partied the night before had clearly been sobered by twenty-three and a half miles on the road.

Six o'clock was the magic hour when the route closed and the mess hall opened, so everyone had to be back by then. Other than those still walking the last two miles to finish, everyone still on the trail was picked up by vans and driven to camp.

As she watched the faces of the weary, Emmy considered how important it was to train for the Walk. She had been lucky. She had found her team early, benefited by a plan that built up endurance and speed, and trained under a leader who understood how to do it. She was also fortunate to walk with friends every step of the way.

As she was about to turn away, she spotted Lauren marching toward the gate. A bright smile lit her pale face, but Alex and Darla walked close beside her. Emmy held up a palm and Lauren slapped it as she entered camp.

"Way to go, girl!" Kat yelled.

Even though Lauren looked happy, it was obvious she was exhausted. When would she crack?

Emmy felt a tap on her shoulder. It was David.

"We're gonna get dinner," he said.

Emmy and Kat joined him and the others and they moved swiftly through the mess line. Her paper plate was loaded up with steaming spaghetti, limp vegetables, and garlic bread. It didn't look appetizing at all, but once she was seated at a long table with the others, she wolfed it down like the last supper.

After dinner, she joined Kat for a massage, groaning with pleasure as her legs were worked to jello. The band was warming up, so they snagged some water and found a place to sit. A man from Pallotta took the microphone and announced that the total number of walkers was three thousand and sixteen, supported by a crew of five hundred and ninety-one. The applause was overwhelming.

Emmy swiveled her head to get a panoramic view of the sea of bodies. It was amazing. There was simply no other word to describe it. So many people all gathered for one reason. She swallowed hard.

"Day Two," boomed the speaker, "is a short, sixteen mile walk." A cheer rippled through the dining tent. As it died away, someone—it sounded suspiciously like Tom—yelled out: "Tell 'em about the hill!"

The announcer laughed and grudgingly admitted: "There *might* be a hill."

Kat turned to Emmy. "Might?" she exclaimed. "Geez!"

The band was okay, but they felt exhausted and headed back to the infield. Emerging from the tunnel, they saw a mass of blue tents billowing across the meadow. It was beautiful. They spotted several team members sitting around the opening to David's tent, so they joined them in conversation.

The sun went down behind the racetrack, twilight settling over them, a soft breeze playing across the field. The smell of the grassy earth and fresh air blended with the sound of soft conversation and laughter, a heady mixture that started closing eyes.

"I have to go to bed," Emmy mumbled.

David smiled. "We should all get some sleep."

"Goodnight" echoed through the group as Emmy and Kat headed back to their tent. They climbed inside and Emmy zipped it up. Taking off her shoes, she placed them next to the flashlight by the entrance, then crawled into her sleeping bag. She wrapped the warm down around herself and stretched out her stiff legs.

"Nine o'clock!" It was a crew member with a megaphone. "Please turn off your radios. Please keep noise to a minimum."

Closing her eyes, she started to drift off. A burst of laughter jolted her awake. It was Tom. He tried to get his chuckle under control, but it erupted into a loud guffaw.

"Oh, for the love of Mike!" a woman shouted. "It's *him* again! Enough already!"

There was dead silence, then Emmy started to giggle and it infected Kat. Soon, laughter rippled through their whole end of camp. It lasted for several minutes and then tapered off into silence. Emmy snuggled back down into her sleeping bag, tired and relieved.

Day One was complete.

Nothing but good stuff ahead.

34

Day Two

Saturday, July 28

In the blackness, Emmy heard the rip of a zipper. Someone grabbed her foot and shook it. She raised her leg to kick and pain ripped through her hamstring. It tightened like a coiled spring and she was instantly awake, crying out in pain.

"Shhh!"

Her foot contracted. Gritting her teeth, she forced the leg to stretch out straight, then pulled herself upright with her stomach to massage the hammy. *God! Geez!* Curling her toes, she stretched her foot to relax it. Kat ruffled around on the other side of the tent.

"What's up?" she asked.

"Keep it quiet," Marianne whispered. "You guys want to clean up in a real bathroom?"

"Uh huh," Kat replied.

"Get your stuff together. We'll be waiting at the tunnel."

Emmy flexed her leg several times. Bolts of pain rushed through her. She was afraid of moving it, but she had to go. Flexing her foot back and forth, she worked to relax the cramps.

"Hustle up," Kat said.

Using the flashlight, they gathered up what they needed. Emmy ripped the pink shirt from the Behemoth. Kat crawled outside as Emmy slipped into her running shoes without tying the laces. She limped along behind Kat to catch up to the others. Marianne led them through the tunnel, an unmarked door, and up onto a patio under the grandstand. She stopped at a door marked "Women." A *real* restroom.

Large mirrors lined the wall above the sinks and everyone grabbed a spot. Quickly, Emmy washed up and dressed. Her leg ached. If she couldn't walk, what would she do? It hurt and every minute it hurt more.

She lifted her memorial shirt with Amy's picture on the back. Kat watched as she held it up and read the imprint.

AMELIA FLEMING

October 20, 1959 - April 16, 2000

There was something in Kat's eyes that she'd never seen before. Surprise? Shock? The date. *That must be it.* Barely three months had passed since the anniversary of her death. There were the signatures of Dan, Annie, Ben, and everyone else flowing around the name and dates. It would be nice to just put it away, but she had promised Barb she'd wear it, so she would.

She would give Amy this one day.

She pulled it over her head, then straightened the arms and smoothed it out. Turning back to her bag, she got out her 3-Day bandana. Folding it into a triangle, she looped it over the top of her head and knotted it beneath her ponytail. She adjusted it so the yellow star showed in the very center of her forehead.

Just like David.

Gathering up her clothing and ditty bag, she turned and hobbled outside, with Kat right behind her. Leaning on the rail, they gazed across the manicured soil of the race track at several thousand blue tents huddled together on the infield. The sky was pale blue.

"I didn't know," Kat said. "I kind of suspected, but didn't know for sure. Who was she?" She nodded at the shirt.

"My aunt," Emmy replied. "She was an artist, pretty famous. I'm surprised you didn't read about it when she died."

"Geez! Of course!"

Emmy smiled at her, but Kat gazed steadily into her eyes, then rested a hand on her hip and sighed.

"It isn't real yet, is it? You haven't accepted it, have you?"

"Sure," Emmy answered.

Kat's lips twitched and she raised an eyebrow. *She doesn't believe me!* Emmy barked out a laugh and tried to smile more brightly.

"I'm okay," she said. "Don't worry."

Turning, Kat leaned down to the rail. Resting her chin on her palm, she gazed wistfully out across the racetrack. Emmy knew the look. Stepping closer, she rested her hand on Kat's shoulder.

"Who was it?" she asked.

"*My* aunt," Kat said. "Jingyi. Four years ago."

She stared out across the tent city with moist eyes. Kat was always so carefree—it was weird to see her sad.

The restrooms emptied out and they trekked back through the tunnel to their tents. Her leg still hurt, but she was starting to work it out. They packed their duffel bags and tent as the sky grew lighter by the minute. More people stirred and the camp began to buzz to life.

The team met up at the tunnel and walked together to turn in their tents and luggage. At six o'clock, they were in line at the mess tent, Emmy still limping. The smell of hot food woke her up and she took a little of everything on her plate.

As they looked for a place to sit, Tom glanced over at her.

"No biscuits and gravy," he said in a forlorn voice.

"You'll live," Kat muttered.

Emmy felt ravished and ate all of her breakfast. David stepped away while she was shoveling food and returned a moment later just as she pushed her plate aside.

"Charley horse?" he asked. Tears rose to her eyes, but she blinked them away, nodding. "Here," he said, unraveling an Ace bandage. He wrapped it tightly around her leg and patted it closed.

She swallowed. He was still looking after her.

"Thanks, David," she muttered, barely getting it out.

Everyone was excited about the day's walk, but it all felt wrong to Emmy: the aching leg, wearing the damned shirt, thinking about Amy. She glanced up at the sky. Bright red streaks of sunlight fired across the treetops.

She felt antsy and had to move, had to test her leg out. The tent filled with people, so she pushed herself up, dumped her tray, and pushed off toward the front gate of the race track. The team was right behind her.

They were not the first ones to arrive at the starting line, but there were only five others ahead of them, a stark contrast to the previous day. Emmy stretched her leg hard and the hammy loosened up. In minutes, it felt good enough to go.

David always knows what to do.

Pacing back and forth, she shook her arms to stay loose. Turning around, she caught someone staring at her shirt. The woman quickly looked away, but Emmy saw clearly the pity on her face and flushed with an old anger.

The last thing I need is pity. I need to walk.

The safety monitor stepped forward and declared the route open. The gate swung wide and everyone surged forward. As was his habit, David started them out at three miles an hour. Normally, Emmy didn't mind the warm-up, but other walkers pulled out ahead of them and Emmy yearned for that speed. She wanted to fly like the wind instead of *slowly* picking up speed. David must have felt it, too, because in a moment, he kicked it into gear and suddenly they *were* flying down the sidewalk.

As they sped along, Emmy's brain shut down. The cheering and honking on the side of the road seemed far away. Businesses, houses, and cars passed in a blur. Even her teammates disappeared. Her breathing was in a perfect rhythm and it was all that existed in the universe. When they took a brief break, she stretched and hydrated, as required, but couldn't talk to anyone.

She felt hollow inside, her thoughts echoing back and forth. The emptiness thrummed and roared and she didn't care. She didn't care about anything. Life had stopped, even as it rushed on, up a little incline that felt flat. They were moving up into the foothills. Somewhere to the west, the Peninsula ridgeline loomed over her.

At ten-thirty, they rolled into the lunch stop. The crew was still setting it up in a large park, so they had to wait. David led them to a tree along an embankment that offered generous shade. The others dropped to the grass, but Emmy stood, looking out into the street, breathing deeply. She was coated in sweat. Her shirt was wet in the back, the armpits, and around the collar. The bandana covering her head was completely soaked. She pulled it off and wrung it out, watching sweat stream into the grass.

Sitting down, she rinsed it with fresh water from her bottle, then flattened it out and set it aside to see if the breeze would dry it. Leaning back, she rested her head against the cool grass of the embankment. The world was blotched with dark streaks. As she studied them in detail, she realized that her sunglasses were covered with little rills of dried sweat. She took them off and looked up at the leafy green canopy rising into the pale blue sky.

Why do I feel so hollow?

For seven months, she had been looking forward to the 3-Day, but now, all she wanted was to die right there, in that moment, lying on the grassy slope with the sun slanting through the trees. She closed her eyes and time streamed past her in a blur.

"Okay," David said. "They're serving lunch."

She listened as those around her pulled themselves up and sauntered away, then a shadow fell across her face.

"Let's go," Kat said.

Opening her eyes, Emmy looked up.

"I need to rest for a minute," she said.

"Nope," Kat replied, extending her hand. "You know what happens when you lay around. Tight muscles. Got a big hill. Can't have tight muscles. Give me your hand." Emmy didn't move. "Hey," Kat said, "have I ever steered you wrong?"

"No."

"Okay, then. Hold out your hand."

Reluctantly, Emmy reached out and they grasped each other's forearm. She planted her feet on the grass and pushed herself up as Kat pulled. When they stood face to face, Kat grinned.

"Atta girl! Let's eat."

They walked out of the dappled shade and into the sun. Emmy put her glasses back on, sweat streaks and all. They strolled through the bodies now flooding the field and up to the chow line. She took her box lunch and they headed back to the tree.

"Big surprise," Kat announced when she opened her box. "Sandwich, chips, fruit, cookie. You'd think they'd at least slip in a Ding Dong or something."

Even though the meal was unsurprising, it was still welcome and they finished every bite. Emmy felt a real flow of gratitude to Kat for rousing her from the grass. She'd never had a girlfriend before who really cared about her. She felt lucky—lucky in so many ways she couldn't even begin to count them all. And suddenly she felt like crying. Even though she couldn't. *I won't.*

The hill was next and it was time to get busy. She splashed water on her sunglasses and dried them on her shirt. She struggled to get the doo-rag on without a mirror.

Turning to Kat, she asked, "How's it look?"

"It's crooked," Kat answered with a smile. "Let me help." She worked at it for a minute. "There. You're fine now."

David and Marianne were seriously stretching, so the two girls joined them and the whole group stretched with controlled intensity.

The hill waited for them and it was time to go to work. No one spoke and Emmy felt the devotion deep inside. At least twenty walkers passed the team as they worked their muscles.

Then a tall, strong black woman strode across the field, her eyes shimmering. She stalked past the team and got on the sidewalk alone. Michael watched her for a moment, then turned to the others with a wicked grin.

"Show time!"

Emmy picked up her water and Gatorade and David and Tom led the way up the embankment. Marianne and Janet followed. Emmy and Kat got in behind them and the rest of the team sorted itself out to walk in pairs.

The route took them farther north, then they turned west and headed up the hill. The incline was shallow at first, but the angle soon pitched upward toward thirty-five degrees. It was a lazy, winding route, but steadily uphill. At first, there weren't many people cheering, but as they worked their way upwards, Emmy saw homes decorated especially for the 3-Day walkers. Large signs were mounted on lawns, bunting was strung along windows, and there was a steady stream of applause and cheering.

Soon, she approached a lamp post with a large sign that read:

"Welcome to Hope Hill!"

Ha! It had to be a joke. Hope was a children's exercise that had no place in the real world. Everyone hoped. Emmy had hoped. Her mother had prayed for months on end. *Lot of good that did.*

She imagined Barb.

Hopeful Activity #768: Hope Hill.

In a driveway up ahead, three kids stood behind a table, holding out paper cups of lemonade. Emmy watched those up ahead of her thank the kids and walk on without taking the offered drinks. The kids looked disappointed, so she stopped and gazed into the face of a little girl, no more than five years old. Her hair was dark blond, cut shoulder length. Large blue eyes, open wide, stared up as her little hand held out a cup. Emmy couldn't resist. Shifting her Gatorade onto her left wrist, she took the cup and downed it in one swallow.

"Mm," she said. "Thanks!"

A wide smile broke across the girl's face and Emmy felt a terrible longing spring up inside, so powerful it hurt. Maybe, if things worked out, she might become a mother herself. But would Barb certify her fit for motherhood? The woman was so tenacious—always a new project no matter how good Emmy felt. On the other hand, Emmy felt very unfit this morning. In fact, she felt more like a child herself.

But Ross would make a good father.

Ross! Shit! She had promised she'd call him the first night, but then completely forgot. *Geez!* She hadn't even turned on her phone since leaving home the previous morning. It rested, inert, inside the Minnow at her belly.

I'll call at the next break. Wow.

She wanted to linger with the child, but they had to move on. Crushing the cup in her hand, she tossed it in the wastebasket. Kat grinned and they returned their attention to the hill, working hard to make up lost ground. The push felt good. Her hammy was totally loose now and both of her legs felt incredibly strong.

"Janice!" It was David's voice, up ahead.

Looking up, she saw David and Tom throw their arms around a middle-aged woman who stood beside a table. Tom laughed and clapped her on the back. When the two men stepped away, Emmy's breath caught in her throat. Janice had dark red hair and large hoop earrings and she looked just like Amy. *Geez!*

"You're not walking this year?" Tom asked.

"No," Janice replied. "This year, I'm just a supporter. You have no idea how hard it was to walk right by my front door up this damned hill!" They all laughed.

She reached into a cooler on the table and pulled out two single grape popsicles. As they hit the air, a thin shell of white frost formed on each one. She handed them to Tom and David, then brought out more and passed them to Janet and Marianne.

Emmy's mouth watered and she suddenly felt the heat. She and Kat stepped up to the table and Janice gave them their own popsicles. She stuck hers in her mouth and the sweet, juicy frozen water tasted simply amazing.

"Turn around," Janice said to them. "Take a look at how far you've come."

It was an awesome view. San Francisco Bay stretched out panoramically behind the airport. In the distance, Mount Diablo loomed over the hills of the East Bay against the horizon. In the sky above, a 747 banked and began its descent to the airport.

"Well, that puts things in perspective," Tom said.

Emmy turned back to face them, but all she saw was Janice, who had been staring at the picture of Amy on the back of her shirt. Her eyes traveled down and she read the name and dates of Amy's life, then looked up into Emmy's eyes. There was no pity, but Emmy felt there was a shared understanding.

"Yes," David replied, nodding at the silent interchange. "Well, we still have a long way to go."

"Stay warm tonight!" Janice said. Emmy nodded.

They continued on up the hill, slurping their popsicles as they climbed. Emmy sucked with a vengeance, completely licking her wooden stick dry. As she put it away in the Minnow for later disposal, she felt a twinge in her back. It was low around the hips, right where it always lived deep into a walk.

She focussed on her rhythm and breathing. All she had to do was keep working. Up and up she went, forever and ever it seemed, ever upward, always upward. The pain in her back worked into her legs with each step, but she kept in rhythm.

Just another hill. I've done it a hundred times before and I'll do it a hundred times again.

She heard cheering, up ahead in the distance. It came from the top of the hill. That was her goal and she was nearly there. On she drove, pushing harder and harder until at last she topped out. The crew clapped and cheered, giving the team high-fives as they caught their breath. Emmy turned to look down the hill. It was a long, long mother and she felt grateful it was done, but the pain in her back required immediate attention.

There was a Grab 'N Go across the street, so she dumped her empty bottles and picked up fresh ones while David began to stretch. A car was parked near the little tent, so she decided to borrow it for a moment. Bracing her hands on the fender, she stretched both legs out behind her and lowered her stomach toward the pavement. As she hung there, Kat moved next to her and took the same position, just as they had done during the sim. A minute later, they pushed themselves back up and sighed with relief.

"Neat trick," Kat chuckled.

After stretching, David strolled past them and the team fell in behind him.

Now that the hill was finished, it was just a matter of getting into camp. They walked down a long block, crossed under Interstate 280 and emerged onto the San Andreas Trail. They were nowhere near the ridgeline, which towered black above them to the west, San Andreas Lake spread out below. It felt really easy now and a few more miles melted away.

There was a Pit Stop up ahead, but there were walkers hanging out at the gate that led to the route along the highway. It was blocked by two crew members. David and Tom walked up front and Emmy followed.

"What's going on?" David asked.

"They're still setting up camp," a crewman answered. "They told us not to let any walkers go till it's ready."

"How long?"

"Not sure. Could be an hour."

"You've got to be kidding!" Tom cried.

Emmy's heart sank. It would be more than an hour. They would all sit around and their muscles would tighten up. A mob would build up behind them and camp would be crowded from the get go. Tom turned away in disgust. David and Emmy followed him back.

"They're not letting anyone through till camp's set up," Tom announced. "Could be an hour."

Marianne looked up at him. "Geez, that sucks. We didn't have that last year."

"Looks like we get to relax for a little while," David said. "Have a snack, hydrate, use the port-o-potties, play games—I don't care, but try not to sleep."

"We should keep a few people up by the gate, holding a place for us," Marianne said. "We can switch off."

"Good idea," David replied. "I'll go first."

"Me, too," Tom added. Joy and Ellen held up their hands, then others did, too. David looked at them and smiled.

"Four should be plenty."

They left and the others fell to the grass. Emmy looked around, uncertain what to do, then she remembered. *Ross! I've got to call him.* The lake looked placid so she wandered down toward it and found a place to sit. When her cell powered up, she had five messages, so she dialed in to get them.

Ross had called last night, wondering how she was doing. Tina wanted to know when the Closing Ceremony started. Her mom had called, offering encouragement. The whole family was coming to the Closing Ceremony.

So much was happening. *Too much.*

It was going to be crazy when the Walk was over. She didn't want it to end, but it had to end. She had to get back to her life, to find a place and move in with Ross, to furnish and decorate—to settle down, finally.

She tabbed the next message.

"Emmy, it's Ross. I hope you're okay. I was really hoping to hear something by now. I'll try to find you this afternoon, so if you get this message, please give me a call."

The urgency in his voice was electric. She had to call him, but there was one more message. She tabbed it.

"Ross again. Listen, I'm up here at Skyline College, waiting for you to get into camp. It's about ten after one. I'll see you soon!"

She punched his speed dial and he picked up first ring.

"Emmy!"

"Ross! God, I'm so sorry I didn't call. I completely forgot about the phone. I hadn't even turned it on!"

He laughed. "Well, you've been busy. Are you okay?"

"I'm fine."

"Where are you?"

"Up around San Andreas Lake. They stopped us because camp's not set up yet."

"Okay, I'll be waiting when you get here."

"Ross?"

"Yes?"

"I love you."

"I love you, too."

She clicked off the phone, burning inside, like a fiery tornado sucking up everything around her.

"I love you." *Famous last words*.

Emmy cocked her head. She always said that to herself. Famous last words: I love you. Why? Where the hell did it come from?

Sitting alone, she stared out across the lake as a bird skimmed the surface, crying out in the thick afternoon air. Time stood still. Everything felt connected, but she still didn't know how "I love you" had become famous last words.

It seemed so close she could almost touch it, but... How?

How?

35

When the gate opened, there was no time to waste. She could hardly breathe. Kicking into top speed, the team moved briskly down along the highway, two by two. Emmy and Kat paced each other, but they didn't talk. It was fast and exhilarating.

They sped down a long hill, then upward, under towering eucalyptus trees. Turning left onto College Drive, they continued uphill past a large suburban area. It took forever. Breathless, they pushed up the hill and there was the crew cheering for them at the entrance of Skyline College.

Ross stood at the back of the receiving line, clapping and cheering. He shook David's hand and slapped high fives with the others. Emmy worked her way through the tunnel of bodies, slapping hands, then sprinted to him and leaped into his arms. She kissed him madly and he whirled her around, laughing.

Inexplicably, she realized, Ross was now everything to her. *Everything!* She gripped him tightly, as tight as a grape popsicle with a frozen white shell.

Kat waited, but not for long.

"Hey, Ross," she said.

"Hi, Kat!" he answered, "Can you take a picture of us?"

"Sure."

Emmy handed over the camera and they posed. *This is for Barb*, she thought. *I've got the shirt, Ross, and a smile. Barb should be happy.*

She had to make Barb happy, no matter what.

"I've got to run get our tent." Kat said as she handed the camera back.

"I'll be right along," Emmy answered.

When Kat turned away, she kissed him again, deeply, as if it was their last kiss, but people were watching. She heard the sniggers, so she finally broke away.

"Gotta help Kat," she said.

"I know. I'll see you tomorrow."

"I'll be there."

She trotted up the sidewalk.

Skyline College sat on a hillside oval, with buildings clustered at the back, perched right along a dip in the ridgeline. Athletic fields massed in front, already blooming with tents. She grabbed the Behemoth and found Kat. They set up the tent, then headed to the main camp.

In the shower truck, she peeled off the memorial shirt and tossed it down on the bench. The picture of Amy stared back at her. It was from Amy's fortieth birthday party. Her hair looked great, but it was a red wig. She wanted to look like herself. *That sounds so weird.* She wanted everything to look normal, even though it would never be normal again. *I think she knew it.* She looked happy that day. How could she possibly have been happy? There was only one road and she was barreling down it with no brakes.

Emmy sighed.

It's time to end Amy's day, the one day I gave her.

Unclasping her necklace, she draped the garnet heart on the shirt so it rested on Amy's throat. *It belongs there. Dad left. She left. How appropriate. She can have it.*

Kat watched from her shower stall. After a moment, she murmured, "Hey, there's a line outside."

Emmy stepped into the hot water. It pounded against her skin, but even as she closed her eyes, she knew that Amy was staring back at her from the bench.

When she was dry, Emmy took the shirt and necklace together and stuffed the bundle into her plastic laundry bag. She dressed, but it felt strange to be without her necklace.

Should I put it back on? Why did I take it off?

Maybe I need to be through with all of this.

Maybe that's how I break free.

The next few hours were dizzy and strange. Moments melted one into the other without the seams that should separate them. She glanced at her watch. It was nearly five o'clock and all she remembered were colors, the turn of legs on bright green grass, the pull of hamstrings bending down, the taste of banana.

Time.

So many people, so much pink. She walked along the sidewalk with Kat after cheering and clapping for incoming walkers.

She felt pumped so full that she could hardly move.

"I have to talk to David," Kat said. "I'll see you later."

She broke away, jogging up the path. Emmy stood for a moment, an island in a tangle of moving bodies. Unsure what to do, she took a step forward, then another. She walked alone and it felt strangely right.

It was a warm, sunny afternoon. She wondered if the legendary fog—that fog so cold (in Tom's words) *it'll freeze your shorts off—*

would come rolling in. A strong marine push could erupt in a heartbeat. Up the road, the ridgeline perched at the back of the college. She considered walking up to take a look.

Like I really need to climb another hill.

With a sigh, she began to work her way upward through the parking lot. The sky was milky in the west. She pushed higher and higher. A low stone wall marked the ridgeline and there it was before her: dense, massive fog. It covered the ocean and all of the city of Pacifica, sprawled out below her on the shore. And it was moving fast. In about an hour, it would envelope camp.

Sitting on the low, stone wall, she watched the tightly packed moisture flow steadily toward her. It felt like her entire life—eighteen years of heaving turbulence—was rushing to break over her. As a girl, she had always colored inside the lines. It was Amy's hand guiding the crayon in a wide arc beyond the controlled form, that opened her eyes to all she couldn't see in the picture.

Abstract. Concrete. Does it matter?

I buried her as if she never existed. I walk inside the lines as if she isn't here, but she is here, now. She wanted to crush the feeling, but it overpowered her.

The fog rolled up the shoreline. Wisps of swirling gray smothered the beach and slipped up the hill, the tentacles of some ancient sea beast, eating Pacifica. The gray monster willed itself to her, tendrils slithering up the side of the mountain, oozing toward her feet.

Abruptly, a cold blast of wind hit her. She jumped. Deep shivers washed over her as freezing cold penetrated her shorts and tee shirt and lifted the hair on her arms, creeping up goosebumps. She had been wrong about the fog—it wouldn't arrive in an hour—

It's here now.

Standing abruptly, she jogged back down the hill to camp, hustling straight to the tent.

Zipping the flap behind her, she struggled out of her running shorts and into a pair of jeans, then pulled on her thermal pants and windbreaker. It was already time for dinner so she hurried to the main camp.

The large, white dining tent rippled in the wind. Gusts of fog flew overhead. Across the grass, the medical tent overflowed with injured walkers, blurry in the haze, shadowy bodies slabbed on tables with dangling IVs.

Crew members were unrolling the side flaps of the mess tent, tying them to the poles with ropes as they buffeted in the wind like sails. Emmy plunged on through the streaming mass of bodies until she spotted David and the others huddled together against the cold. Angling over, she slipped into the circle.

"There you are!" David said. "You ready for our last dinner?"

Thousands of zombies scrambled around them in the violent cloud. Wind whipped droplets of dew like ice, splatting against the tent's canvas. They plunged through the flap and worried their way into the chow line. Steam rose from the food as it hit the plate, but when Emmy sat down, it was already cold.

It didn't matter. She looked around the table at faces that had meant so much to her. This was their final dinner together and she didn't want to let go of it. She took photos, one after another, so she would never forget the evening—all of them huddled together, as the wind rattled the tent, blistering their ears so they had to shout.

David, laughing, speared a cold bean on his fork and offered it to Janet. Marianne, wise and beautiful, rested her palm on Kat's shoulder, her smile sad, whimsical. Huddled inside her hoodie, Juliette cringed with chill, her red nose glowing, her eyes laughing at Tom and Michael's prank. Bertina sat like Buddha, enfolded in her jacket.

Emmy wanted to hold onto them so tight. She loved them all. She loved the hours they had spent training together—all of the sweat, the aches, blisters, exhaustion—that unnamed, primal something that clumped them together. She loved them all.

Famous last words.

Emmy shook her head. Once again. "Famous last words." Where on earth did it come from? She felt sick inside. She was about to lose the most important people in her life. And she'd already lost the most important person in her life once. *Not again.*

The band started playing and the team began to drift apart. One by one, the table emptied until Emmy sat alone with David. He drummed his fingers on the table, then looked up at her.

"Well," he said, "I think it's time."

"Time for what?"

"The Memory Tent."

"What's the Memory Tent?"

He leaned into his arm on the table and peered at her. Their eyes were locked across the space between them.

"Every year they set aside a special tent... It gives us—those of us who've lost someone to breast cancer—a chance to write a message to the person we've lost. They have these giant sheets of paper. Then, tomorrow, for the Closing Ceremony, they hang them up so that everyone can read the messages."

He held her eyes, unmoving, as he paused for a moment.

Swallowing hard, she blinked and turned her gaze down at the grass under her stained shoes.

"Anyway," he continued, "I want to write a little note to Joey. Why don't you come along?" She glanced up at him, clenched inside, her muscles locked. She had to say no, but couldn't find the breath. She couldn't move. "You don't have to if you don't want to," he said, "but I'd appreciate the company."

She found his eyes. For some reason, he wanted her there—and she wanted to help him. Could she stand around in a mausoleum while he wrote his note? Could she stand like a statue while he grieved? She owed him. She owed him big time. He was always there for her; now she had to be there for him.

I can do it. Can't I?

She nodded. They stood together and made their way out into the howling night. Shivering ghosts in Nike and Adidas ran to and fro in the thick fog, huddled under silver Mylar blankets. The air was wet and it whipped around them like rain. They tramped through the soggy grass to the entrance. He held the flap open for her. She stepped inside and he followed.

Three long tables crossed the tent, each with sheets of white paper on top, about three feet wide and six feet long. It was surreal, filmy, out of focus. A few ghosts sat huddled around the tables. Women and men hugged each other, sniffling or sobbing. The tent felt swollen with grief and she couldn't bring herself to face it. Her calves tightened like steel. She was ready to run. In fact, she turned, but David put arm his around her shoulder, squeezing. He guided them to an empty space. Pulling out a chair, he sat and picked up a Sharpie. He was perfectly still, thinking about what he was going to write.

How can he do it? How can anyone face that paper?

Her hands gripped his shoulder. He looked up at her, rested his hand on hers for a moment, then turned again to the paper.

Her eyes drifted across the scroll:

Dear Mom,

Thank you SO much for your wisdom. Not a day goes by that I don't think about something you said or did to help us live our lives. I have to say that we are all well and happy, because I know that's the first thing you would ask. We love and miss you so much!

Jane

There was a red heart next to it with the name:

Eleanor Hightower

Eleanor! God, poor Eleanor!

Another ghost on this day of ghosts. Swaying with dizziness, she gripped David's shoulders tightly. Leaning forward, he wrote in large, block letters. She watched intently as he wrote his message.

Dear Joey,

We're still trying to find a cure. I won't rest until we do. Every day, I walk through San Francisco and all I can think of is you. I love you with all my heart and I always will.

Rest in peace, my love.

David

Pushing the chair back, he stood and whipped off his glasses. He didn't sob; he didn't make a sound. Quietly, he wiped the tears from his eyes and then put his glasses back on. When he turned to her, she wrapped her arms around him and held him tightly. She buried her face against his chest and squeezed him. He gripped her for a moment, then patted her on the back.

"Your turn," he said.

"No!" The word was lost in the folds of his jacket. "I can't!"

She had never been so afraid of anything in her life. She stood, frozen in place, but David gently disentangled her. He turned her to the chair and helped her to sit. He shifted the paper to a blank spot next to his message, then lifted the pen and passed it to her.

She took it between her trembling fingers and stared down at the blank space.

"I can't," she said again.

"Yes, you can," he replied, his voice warm, soothing. Fatherly. "You really need to do this, Emmy. You have to do it for yourself. You have to say goodbye."

The words echoed through her.

...to say goodbye...

Something twisted inside, wrenching her back into the room at California Pacific. Amy sat in bed, more ghost than flesh. Emmy stood across the room, staring at her, still absorbing the news that she'd given up the fight.

Amy's voice brought her violently into focus.

"Emmy... We won't see each other again."

It was unacceptable. Emmy stared at her in silence, the blood roaring in her ears. Nothing was acceptable any more. The whole world was unacceptable.

"Come here," Amy said, opening her arms. "I want to say goodbye."

...to say goodbye...

In her panic, Emmy couldn't move. She couldn't go to Amy. She couldn't say goodbye. In a moment of absolute clarity, she now understood that the girl she was a year ago could never accept Amy's death, even though she saw Amy's eyes pleading with her to do it.

"Emmy," Amy had said, "I love you."

Famous last words.

As she sat at the table, the Sharpie trembling in her fingers, she understood. And remembered in horror how she had turned and ran to the door, how she had banged it open and stormed into the hallway, how she had leaned against the cold wall and closed her eyes and blanked it all away, wished it all away, and entered into a world where she was determined to never accept it.

Emmy forced her eyes up from the paper in front of her and stared around the room in panic.

My God, I ran away without saying goodbye!

The full gravity of her action throbbed through her. All Amy had wanted was to hold her one more time, to say goodbye to a beloved niece. And Emmy had turned away, refusing to give comfort and love.

It was an act so cowardly and selfish that she flushed with grief and regret.

"It's okay," David said. "Maybe I pushed you too hard."

Her fingers shook madly above the paper.

Suddenly, she inhaled, a deep, shivering gasp. She blew it out, but another followed. Her heart contracted. All she wanted now was a chance to hold Amy one last time.

Air! I need air!

She sucked it in eagerly. Blood pounded through her body, ripping at her throat. She had to tell Amy! There was only one thing to write. The Sharpie stabbed down onto the paper and she scrawled, her fingers moving on their own, writing:

"I'm sorry!"

She felt another contraction. From deep inside. With every ounce of strength left, she forced her muscles to contain it, but this one soared up, out into the ghostly cold air. It emerged as a thin, ragged whimper.

I can't! I won't!

Gasping, she choked on the wail that was clawing its way out of her. Her eyes were full. She blinked and huge tears squeezed out, rolling down her cheeks, falling on the paper. She sucked in another deep breath and completely lost control, sobbing like dying animal.

Somehow, Kat appeared by her side, stroking her hair. She stood abruptly and the chair tipped over. David wrapped his arms around her and she collapsed into them.

"I'm sorry!" she cried.

Kat wrapped her arm around Emmy and David held both of them. They wept together. Then other arms enfolded them, complete strangers, making a big, warm circle. Emmy cried until she was completely empty and sick inside and then she cried more. And when it finally subsided, she was so weak she could hardly stand. Her eyes were swollen and her nose was running.

After being so full, emptiness engulfed her. She couldn't survive it. *I can't!* But she felt the warmth of those around her, of David and Kat. *They* had survived.

She would survive.

David and Kat walked her back to the tent, each supporting from the side. The fog was so thick they couldn't see six feet in front of them, but Kat knew the way and she guided them forward.

As she unzipped the tent, David held Emmy.

"Sleep it out," he said to her. "Just lie down and let everything melt away."

She sniffled and looked up at him.

"David—"

"It's okay," he said.

Somehow, she bent over and crawled into the dark little tent, with Kat right behind her. She pulled off her shoes and fumbled with the sleeping bag. Kat turned on the flashlight and unzipped the bag for her. She crawled up on her air mattress and pulled the sleeping bag around her. Kat zipped it up so she was snug inside.

She blew out a breath. It would be a different world tomorrow, completely different. She peered through the darkness and tried to see Kat.

"I'm so thankful you're a part of my life," she said.

"I love you, too," Kat answered.

That's how it should be and that's how it is. Period.

It was so cold. The wind ripped against the tent and large drops of fog splashed against it. Curled up in a ball, Emmy radiated and absorbed her own warmth.

And in that warmth, she gave herself over to sleep.

36

Day Three

Sunday, July 29

It hurt. God, but it hurt.

She had to pee so bad she thought she might explode.

I gotta get up.

Wind blasted the tent and splattered droplets of fog against the shell, but she was so hot in her sleeping bag that her hair was matted against her forehead. She tried to open her eyes, but they were swollen shut. *Where's the zipper?* She blinked several times, but just couldn't see.

She pulled the zipper and cold air rushed in. Her legs were stiff as she poked them out. Fumbling at the foot of the tent, she found the flashlight and turned it on. She pulled on her shoes, unzipped the tent flap, and quickly crawled out onto the wet grass. A gust of cold wind battered against her. It hurt to turn around, but she zipped the fly closed. As she forced herself to stand, fresh tears rose to her eyes. The flashlight beam wheeled around camp until it landed on a row of port-o-potties. She hobbled toward them, opened one up, and stepped inside.

Fumbling with her thermal pants, she snapped and zippered her jeans. Somehow she pulled everything down, sat, and let go. She shivered with pure joy. It was the longest pee of her life—and it felt just *wonderful* to let everything go.

As she began to relax, she wondered what had happened the night before. *God, when was the last time I peed?*

Last night. Fog. Dinner. Memory Tent.

Oh, my God, Amy! How could I have done that to you? She felt deeply humiliated—how could she possibly have let Amy down? And all because she was scared.

I cried. God, I cried in front of David and Kat.

And that message... "I'm sorry!" *God, Amy, I'm so sorry!* It was probably written in the shaky hand of a madwoman. Maybe there was still time to fix it.

Her butt was freezing. There was no time like now. Buttoned up against the cold, she pushed out into the wind. The Memory Tent was dark, chilly—much more like a mausoleum now that it was dark and empty. The flashlight beam made the shadows stark and eerie.

She sat, holding the flashlight above the paper. In the circle of light, her writing looked blotchy. "I'm sorry!" It was pathetic. Completely inadequate. How could she have turned her back on Amy? She sniffled. At least she *was* sorry. That was the better part of her at this moment. She had humiliated herself in front of the one woman she loved and revered. And all because she was scared?

I'm not scared now, just humble.

She picked up the pen and began to write. Above her screaming apology, she wrote, "Dear Amy," then continued below it.

"Dr. Jenner was wrong. I have to forgive *myself* because *I* let you down. I won't let you down again. I'll dedicate my life to finding a cure for breast cancer. I'll live my life the very best I can—as you lived yours." She choked and tears flowed from her eyes. She signed it: "Your loving niece, Emmy Wells."

Dashing away the tears, she flipped the Sharpie onto the table. It would be okay now. *I'll be okay.* It was time to get ready. There were more than twenty miles to San Francisco. The shower trailers were just opening, so she picked up the Behemoth and hurried to get clean. She could only imagine how horrid she must look.

When she was clean and dry, she studied herself in the mirror. Her eyes were still puffy and bloodshot, but there was nothing she could do about it. She put on her Team Aquatic Park tee shirt and her team baseball cap, then dug around for her garnet heart and put it back where it belonged—around her neck. She hurried back to the tent. Kat was already awake and dressed.

"How are you?" she asked.

"Okay. I'm sorry about last night."

"Don't be sorry. It was good for you."

"Thanks for being there."

Emmy looked at her. It was amazing that Kat had showed up at the exact time she was needed. Kat glanced at her and then looked away. Maybe it wasn't amazing.

"You knew."

"Don't get mad at me."

Sitting down on her air mattress, Emmy stared at her.

"Mad about what?"

"I asked David to take you to the Memory Tent. I thought it would be good for you."

She turned away. Emmy wasn't at all sure how she felt about it, but she realized Kat was right. *It was good for me.* She couldn't be mad at Kat. As she looked at Kat's hair, she saw a single braid trailing down her back, but it was crooked.

"You've botched your braid," she said. "Can I fix it?"

Kat glanced at her. "Thanks."

Undoing it, she started over. The wind battered the little tent, but it was cozy inside. The quiet time was exactly what she needed. And for once, there was no hurry. The team picture was scheduled for seven o'clock, so, no matter what, they would leave late.

Emmy was fine with it. Having a team picture meant a lot more than sprinting up and down hills and walking like mad all morning. Even with the late start, most of the team should be done by early afternoon. The Closing Ceremony wasn't until five o'clock, so there was no need rush. David had invited them to join him around three o'clock for a Tsingtao and appetizers at a Chinese restaurant near the holding area, so that was the only deadline she was working on.

After breakfast, they wandered over to the photo area. The fog was lifting and the wind had settled down. They waited behind other teams and stretched to keep loose.

When they were called, they arranged themselves into rows, then the photographer moved them around a bit. The first row sat on the soggy grass. David was in the middle, conspicuous in his running shorts—everyone else wore thermals, tights or sweat pants. A second line of people kneeled behind them. Kat and Emmy were there, along with Tom, Marianne, and Janet. Then there was a group of smaller people standing behind them and finally the tallest people formed a line at the back. Almost everyone was smiling or laughing. When the picture was taken, those in the back and on the sides raised their hands, palms open.

Emmy smiled for the camera, but she wasn't feeling it. They were all together for the last time. It was almost over. This was her team. She loved them. She didn't want to let them go.

After the picture, the team scattered. Emmy and Kat joined Tom, Marianne, Janet, Juliette, Joy, Ellen, Michael, Bertina, Rachel, Karen, and Rhonda, all clustered around David. These were her closest friends and she needed to be with them. David turned, picked up water and Gatorade, and walked toward the departing stream of bodies. The team followed along, leaving their final camp behind. Emmy glanced back. She would never forget Skyline College.

The exit took them right into the teeth of the wind. There were large pockets of fog along the rolling hills of the ridgeline. At Skyline Boulevard, the route turned north toward San Francisco. She was going home. Up and down over the rolling hills, they kept a good pace, passing hundreds of people, making up lost time.

Turning west, she entered a residential area. She couldn't really orient herself, but it looked like they were heading back toward the ridgeline. They continued to pass scores of people at such a pace that there was no time for talking. Emmy was fine with it; she didn't even want to think.

Then—down the block—she saw the huge concrete supports that held up the Pacific Coast Highway—the same highway Ross had taken in the Scoupe that day in March—she remembered looking down and wondering if she could ever make it to the top.

Well, here I am. I made it. And it feels damn good!

She passed under the highway and came to the end of the block. To the southwest, the white beaches of Pacifica spread out far below her, all the way to Pedro Point. It was so beautiful that she took a photo to remember this moment.

Turning away was like leaving a part of her behind. The route took them up a little residential street called Skyline Drive—another hill—and a really good one. Kat moved up beside her and they worked it together, just like they had worked the hills of San Francisco for the last seven months.

It felt good. Her sore muscles responded right away. She needed the hill. They passed more and more people on their way up and every step felt good. At the top, they were rewarded with a view of San Francisco, gleaming far off in the distance. The City was within reach now.

After quickly hydrating, they turned their attention to the downslope—and it was a very long way down. It felt like they descended at least half way down the ridgeline. There was a crossover back to the highway, then a break area where everyone on the team switched partners. Juliette teamed up with Emmy.

Leaving the sidewalk behind, they headed out on a trail that led across the bluffs. The Pacific Ocean spread out below them and now Emmy saw the Marin Headlands jutting out of the ocean to the north. The sun broke out above the fog and suddenly they were bathed in bright, warm sunlight. As she eased her way down the bluff, Emmy was struck by the intoxicating smell of salty sea air.

She was almost home.

Routed back to the highway again, they continued on toward San Francisco, moving lower down the ridge. Along the highway, a large sign in the median read:

San Francisco City Limits

Wow! It was amazing. The end was literally in sight. The two girls skipped across to the median and took photos of each other standing in front of the sign. Then they were routed into the Fort Funston parking lot for another break. When they set off again, Tom walked beside her as they tramped along the bluffs.

"Almost home!" he said.

"Yeah," she smiled. "It's gonna be good."

"I can't wait to see Kate again. God, but I miss her!"

"Kate? Your wife?"

"Yes. You've met her, haven't you?"

"Just briefly. At Bay to Breakers."

"I remember," he said. "She's an amazing woman. But she hates the Walk." He sighed and smiled. "She doesn't like to have me gone so much."

"At least it's for a good cause."

"Yeah, she knows that. Remember when I told you about Jessica Timmons? She was a friend of Kate's. So, even though she grumbles about the 'Damned Walk,' she gives me twenty-five dollars every year—out of her personal bank account."

Emmy glanced over at him. "Is Rachel...?"

He nodded. "One of her girls."

She smiled. "I'm glad she's walking."

"You and me both!" He grinned. "Symmetry."

They came over a little knob and walked down the last few feet to the sands of Ocean Beach. She'd never loved it more than she did at that moment. They were so close to Golden Gate Park she could almost touch it. A gentle breeze blew from the Pacific and it felt incredible to walk along and listen to the breakers rolling in.

After about a mile, they came to another break area. Emmy hydrated and stretched while the team reassembled, then Marianne partnered with her for the final few miles to the lunch break in Golden Gate Park. They walked in silence up the beach, but they were both smiling. At Lincoln Way, they crossed over to the park and marched along a soft path into the shade of big, leafy trees.

Then she heard cheering and soon she stepped into a tunnel of crew members slapping hands. To one side, she saw Barb grinning and clapping. She looked like a big kid in a tee shirt and jeans, but Emmy was so glad to see her. Breaking off the path, she stepped directly into a bear hug.

"This is amazing!" Barb cried, thumping her back.

Emmy pulled back and looked into her eyes.

"I've got so much to tell you," she said, but the words choked in her throat and she felt tears coming to her eyes. "So much has happened."

"I see," Barb replied, nodding. *She really does see.* Emmy felt it strongly: Barb knew that something *big* had changed. She reached out to touch Emmy's cheek and her eyes twinkled. "Perhaps we can talk about it on Tuesday?"

"Yes. This is our lunch break."

"I don't want to hold you up."

"Come with me."

Barb tagged along as she picked up her box lunch, then they sat together in the grass while she quickly ate. She tried to explain a little about the route and the Pit Stops along the way, but she saved her experience in the Memory Tent for their next appointment.

It was going to be a *way* interesting conversation.

David and the others began to stretch, so Emmy tried to get up. Rocking back to push up, she felt all of the accumulated pain of fifty miles on the road. *I never should have sat down.* Barb offered her a hand and she took it gratefully.

"How much farther?" Barb asked as she pulled Emmy up.

"Ten miles, more or less."

"Will you make it okay?"

"Oh, yeah. I'm on adrenaline now. That'll see me through." She squeezed Barb's hands. "I've got to stretch."

"Okay," Barb replied. "See you Tuesday."

Emmy worked her sore muscles and breathed the clean air of Golden Gate Park. *So close to the end.* She couldn't believe it was almost over. And now she didn't want it to end. The whole experience had enhanced her life in a thousand little ways and she didn't want to let it go.

Seven months of hard work. One big payoff.

Then, nothing.

Of course, I'll keep walking. David was forming the Aquatic Park Walking Club and she would join them, walking every weekend she could. But there was no question: something would be missing from her life. It would be a big hole that she would have to fill somehow. She could spend more time with her family and friends. There was work and school. Apartment hunting, then moving, furnishing, decorating. Sketching and painting. Not to mention Ross.

Maybe the hole wasn't so big after all.

But next January, she would begin training all over again. Fundraising would be harder next year, but she relished the challenge. *I'll have to change my pitch. My whole approach.*

The team set off across Golden Gate Park, twelve of them now, all walking more or less together, but spread out in pairs. Emmy moved up next to David. She hadn't walked with him all day and just wanted a little time in his company.

The route led them out to Fulton Street, three blocks from her apartment. Three blocks from her bed. Now she understood how Janice felt walking right past her own front door on Hope Hill.

What a trip. Only four days ago, she had left here and rode all the way down the Peninsula. She had walked back. The last four days seemed more like four months. She'd have to write it all down before she forgot the details. Ross wanted details.

David was quiet, concentrating on the street ahead. That was his way. She remembered his message to Joey: "I walk the streets of San Francisco and all I can think about is you."

It was very romantic, but David was a good man and he deserved to be happy. He needed someone to pull him out of his mourning. A good woman. He deserved one. And she knew one—Joanna Ferguson, from work. She was about his age. She was a breast cancer survivor. They'd be perfect for each other. But she wondered how he'd react to having another Joanna in his life.

They turned onto Park Presidio and continued north toward Lake Street. This route was too familiar—it led to a deadly hill.

"David," she said, her voice calm. "You didn't talk them into adding the Pacific Street hill, did you?"

He threw back his head and laughed.

"No, I have no influence on the route, but if it's the same as last year, we'll go up through the Presidio."

She chuckled. "That's bad enough."

When they reached Lake Street, they turned up into the Presidio. There was a Pit Stop in the parking lot of the old Marine hospital, so they picked up fresh hydration and stretched before heading up the hill. It felt more like home with every step.

Kat fell in beside her and they worked the hill together. It was great to have her best friend by her side. And it was wonderful to walk through familiar territory. Her hip joints and feet were fairly well swollen and her back ached, but this was the last hill, so she worked it with Kat, just like always.

They topped out and the route took them up to Immigrant Lookout. The Marin headlands stood stark in the distance, miles across the ocean as it rushed to the Golden Gate. They walked in the shade of tall evergreens and Emmy felt so happy she could cry. This was the San Francisco she loved with all her heart. It was wonderful and amazing and she was fully a part of it.

They passed under Highway 1 and there was the Golden Gate

Bridge on their left, rising up to the sky, another sign of home. Downhill, they passed the national cemetery, then, cutting back, they finally emerged from the Presidio, heading due east into a mass of humanity on Chestnut Street.

Coffee shops and bistros had expanded out onto the sidewalk, compounding traffic and impeding their progress. Some people knew what was going on and they cheered, but others just wanted their morning latte without three thousand walkers trampling through them.

Emmy weaved and dodged around people and tables, but it was exhilarating. Her heart pounded. They were literally within a few short blocks of the end! She passed a pizza parlor with sidewalk seating and the smell fresh from the oven was intoxicating. Momentum carries her past it, but she didn't mind. There was a Tsingtao somewhere down the road with her name on it.

Another intersection and one of the San Jose bicycle cops blocked the way at the corner, routing them across the street, where there was a corridor of crew members cheering. Emmy stepped into the corridor, slapping hands as she walked, emerging into the field of the Moscone Recreation Center. Up in front of her, David yelled as he slapped one hand after another. Emmy whooped and screamed as she strutted up the aisle of crew members.

From the side, Kat hugged her and then others joined in. Juliette wept and Emmy laughed as she pulled her into the hug. The three of them rocked back and forth as tears streamed down Juliette's cheeks. Kat was laughing, too.

"What are you crying for?" she called out.

Juliette looked at them and fought against a sob that was forcing itself over her. "I'm so happy!" she bawled. It was so incongruous that all of them laughed, even as Juliette continued to cry.

37

David waded into the crowd and the team followed him back to a tent into the middle of the field. There were stacks of shirts on the counter. Emmy gave a volunteer her Walker Number.

"What size shirt?" the woman asked.

"Medium."

She pulled a shirt from the stack and passed it over.

"Here you go," she said. "Congratulations!"

Emmy unfolded the shirt. The dark blue, long-sleeved tee was her reward for completing the Walk. The front had the Avon Breast Cancer 3-Day logo stenciled in white, both arms had the word AVON running down the outside, and on the back, printed in large white letters, it read:

July 27th - 29th, 2001
San Jose to San Francisco

It was beautiful!

Juliette pulled off her team tee shirt and shrugged into her blue one, so Emmy did, too. Looking at everyone, she blow out a long, happy breath of air. *We made it.*

"Look!" Juliette said. Emmy turned to face Marianne. Her shirt was pink, with dark blue lettering. Janet and Karen also wore the pink shirts.

"Survivors," Kat said. "The survivors wear pink."

Emmy picked up fresh water and Gatorade, hydrated, used the port-o-potty, then joined her teammates in stretching.

When she bent forward, pain shot through her hamstrings. *Geez, I hurt all over. Didn't even notice till now.* Every movement hurt like hell. She glanced around the large field and saw people stumbling or walking like old ladies. Many had fallen to the grass and weren't moving at all. Emmy wanted to lie down, too, but she couldn't let her muscles tighten up. She stretched again and the ache was too much. It was time to get help. She hobbled to the medical tent. One of the workers looked up at her.

"What's wrong?" she asked.

"Do you have any Motrin?"

"We've got ibuprofen." She smiled, lifted a bottle and shook out two pills.

"Thanks!" Emmy tossed them in her mouth and chugged water,

then returned to the team.

"Who's up for a beer?" David asked.

Smiles broke out all around. He led the way to the back of the field and they quietly slipped out an exit by the tennis courts. They headed south up a little hill. Another hill. For some reason, it made Emmy giggle and she couldn't stop.

"What's so funny?" Tom asked.

"We're going up another hill," she sputtered,. It wasn't funny, really, but everyone caught the mood and guffawed as they struggled up the little incline.

It was worth it. They entered a cool, dark restaurant and a friendly Chinese gentleman escorted them to a table. The general order was Tsingtao, but Janet also ordered five plates of appetizers. Emmy felt like a goofy grin was permanently plastered on her face.

A glass was placed on the table before her and the waiter poured the beer until it had a nice, beautiful head, then put the bottle down beside it. A Chinese girl arrived with more drinks. It was all Emmy could do to keep from tipping up the glass before everyone had their drinks, but finally, they lifted their glasses together.

David grinned as he looked around the group.

"Here's to five-point-five million dollars!"

"Amen!" Marianne cried.

As their arms reached out to clink glasses, everyone repeated the sum, "Five-point-five million!" Emmy gulped almost half the glass and felt a foam mustache on her upper lip. It didn't matter. Tilting the glass down, she licked it off.

Everyone started talking at once. She sat back and watched as the conversation wandered all over the place. Everyone was giddy and their laughter was loud and a little crazy.

I'll never forget how good this feels. If I do the 3-Day for the rest of my life, nothing will ever top this.

Standing up painfully, she stepped back and took a photo. Others wanted pictures, too, so they posed over and over again, then the Chinese waiter took pictures of the group.

The waitress arrived with appetizers and there was a flurry of forks and chopsticks as they dug in. Emmy snagged a spring roll and dipped it in sweet pepper sauce. After blowing on it for a moment, she lifted it to her mouth and bit off the entire end. Juices squished out on her chin and she leaned over the saucer. Laughing, Kat applied a napkin to her face. *God, but it's good!* She stabbed a pot sticker and squeezed hot mustard on it. *So good!*

It was four o'clock when they made their way back to the holding area, which had turned festive. Complete strangers hugged each other and laughter soared back and forth across the field. Emmy followed Kat up to the welcoming corridor and they cheered the walkers still coming in.

Shortly after they arrived, Lauren hobbled up the line, with Alex and Darla holding her up. Her smile was angelic and her eyes were bright with tears. Emmy screamed and clapped, then threw her arms around Lauren. Together, they stumbled back to the field and collapsed to the ground. Lying on her back, Lauren laughed and cried at the same time.

Emmy helped her up and pointed to the check-in tent, then joined Kat. She was getting hoarse from all the cheering, so she had to stop. The last of the walkers trickled in and then the San Jose Police pedaled in on their bicycles and everyone cheered wildly. Last of all, the vans pulled up with those who couldn't finish in time, but they were cheered as if they had finished every mile of the Walk. They were entitled to it. They had earned it.

Lauren, Marianne, Karen, and Janet were summoned to the opposite end of the field. All of the survivors, in their pink shirts, moved there together.

"Follow me," David said. The team fell in behind the group

forming at the back gate and waited for fifteen minutes before they finally start moving.

The streets were closed so they walked four and five abreast onto Cervantes Boulevard, a long, diagonal street that took them all the way down to Marina Green. A crowd of people cheered and horns honked continuously.

As they walked along, Juliette looked like she was about to cry again, so Emmy put her arm around her. Kat held her from the other side and the three of them walked together, hugging. It was nearly half a mile to the Marina Green and it hurt every step of the way, but they no longer cared about the pain.

When they arrived, the crowd was enormous. At the other end of the Green, a stage had been erected. The walkers were hustled through an entrance and Emmy heard the swelling of music, then a man's voice, echoing through gigantic speakers, yelling a welcome to "the three thousand walkers of the San Francisco Avon Breast Cancer 3-Day."

A massive cheer went up from the crowd. David and Tom raised their fists in the air, so Juliette, Kat, and Emmy raised their own clenched hands together.

As she walked toward the stage, Emmy looked for her friends and family, but there were so many people she couldn't distinguish individuals. They surged forward, a massive sea of dark blue shirts. The cheering and the music continued and Juliette wept again. Kat was crying, too, but Emmy was just so happy she couldn't stop grinning.

A woman stepped up to the microphone at the podium and urged a welcome to the breast cancer survivors. Another cheer erupted. Emmy found her hoarse voice and joined the others in crying out. A swell of pink shirts erupted into the sea of blue as the survivors entered the arena. Emmy picked out her friends, lifting their joined hands in the air.

It was chaos for a few minutes and when it settled down, the woman on stage called forth the circle of survivors from the very first morning. It was quiet as the women walked forward, holding hands to form the empty space that represented the spirit of all of those who had died from breast cancer. The circle held Amy's spirit, too. For the first time since early morning, when she finished writing her message, Emmy opened up and wept for her. There would never be a more fitting memorial than the circle.

A man stepped to the microphone and introduced the crew. Before he finished, the cheers drowned him out as crew members wearing white, long sleeved tee shirts flooded the elevated walkways. The noise was so loud it filled the shoreline.

Around her, Emmy saw walkers holding shoes in the air, so she kneeled and quickly slid off her right shoe and held it high. Her ears rang with thousands of voices. At last the cacophony subsided and the man on the stage gave a stirring speech as music swelled through the gigantic speakers. "This is not an ending," he cried in a hoarse voice. "Let this be a beginning!"

Emmy screamed again, adding what was left of her voice to the thousands around her. The music swelled to a crescendo and the cheering grew even louder. Everyone jumped around and screamed, stabbing their shoes high in the air. Gradually, the barricades fell and the noise subsided.

Emmy was limp from exhaustion.

Arms wrapped around her and she moved from person to person as they hugged their way toward the spectators. Bit by bit, the crowd dissipated around them. David gathered her into his arms and she held him tight for a long moment.

"Let's go find our families," he rasped.

They trudged through the mass of bodies. Kat saw her family first and turned to Emmy.

"Lunch Wednesday?"

"The Wok?"

"Eleven forty-five! See you there!"

Kat trotted away from their little group and fell into her father's arms. Karen spotted her husband, so she and Rhonda broke away. One by one, Emmy watched her friends disappear into the crowd. She was walking alone with David when she spotted Grace jumping up and down and waving her arms over her head.

A rush of joy hit her and she turned to David.

"I've got to go."

"I know," he replied, "I'll call you when we schedule the first club walk. Go see your family." He smiled.

Grace plunged through the crowd with Jill right behind her. All at once, everyone converged on Emmy, even her brother Dean. She hugged everyone, then Tina and Joanna joined them. When Emmy looked up, tears ran from Dean's eyes and she hugged him tighter. She turned around and Ross snapped a picture of them. Everyone talked at once and she couldn't understand what anyone was saying.

Turning around, she looked for David and spotted him with his family. It was over.

It was really and truly over.

She turned back to her family and Ross folded her into his arms, holding her tight. Her mother was crying, so she pulled away from

Ross and hugged her, too.

"I've got us reservations at McCormick and Kuleto's," Ross said. "We can talk there."

"I've got to get the Behemoth," Emmy said.

"The Behemoth?"

"Long story. Tell you later."

They headed toward the trucks. The adrenaline that had carried her through the afternoon was gone and her legs and feet hurt so bad she could hardly walk. Ross slipped his arm around her and helped her along. When she found the Behemoth, she opened it and pulled out a pair of jeans, slipping them on over her running shorts.

She and Ross rode with her family, while Tina and Joanna took Tina's car through the snarled traffic. Exhaustion was claiming her bit by bit. Walking up the steps to the restaurant felt unbearable. There were a thousand questions about the Walk and she answered them as best she could, croaking away with her hoarse voice. While everyone else ate dinner, Emmy simply ordered coffee and vanilla ice cream with strawberries.

The caffeine gave her a little kick, but she was dreading tomorrow. It would be hell to get out of bed.

Afterward, her mother dropped them off to pick up the Scoupe at

Fort Mason. Ross helped her into the car and helped her out when they got back to his apartment. She drew a very hot bath, took two Motrin, and fell asleep in the tub. After a while, Ross woke her, dried her, and practically carried her to bed. She didn't even want to think about pajamas, so she crawled naked between the sheets. Sitting on the edge of the bed, he held her hand.

She didn't want to let go of him. Her mind tumbled around as she thought about the last four days. Out of it all, she saw Hope Hill. *At the end of the day, there has to be hope.* She prayed that their footsteps would pave the way to find a cure, so that other incredible people, like Amelia Fleming, could live out their lives in peace.

The fight against breast cancer is a long walk. It's a walk against time that should end in a great shout of joy with everyone holding their shoes to the sky.

Ross leaned down and gently kissed her lips.

And she took that promise to rest.

Afterward

Friday, April 16, 2010

Emmy McMahon sat on a bench near the grave of Amelia Fleming. The site afforded a beautiful view of San Bruno Mountain just a few miles to the east. She sat quietly, admiring the beautiful flowers surrounding the headstone, deeply inhaling the crisp, clean air of morning.

It was her yearly pilgrimage. Nine years in a row she had taken this day for herself. She didn't work. She didn't walk. And she didn't play. It was the one day she gave herself over to sorrow. There was a time for death and a time for life and she made the distinction a clean one.

The kids were in school, which was good. She was always glad when April 16th happened on a school day. She didn't like to involve the children in her grief. They'd been lucky so far—no funerals in their young lives. They would eventually have to face death, but she still had time to prepare them for it.

Sadly, she had become an expert on the topic.

A little part of her died every time she thought of Amy. Or of Lauren Sheridan and Karen Miller. All lost to breast cancer.

Emmy closed her eyes and curled her arms around herself. When Lauren had died in 2003, they all knew it was coming. No surprise—not easy, but preparation is everything.

Karen's death had hit fast and hard. She was one of the Pacific Six, the six women who had dragged themselves up the Pacific Street hill on the last day of the training sim in 2001. It had been only seven weeks and four days from diagnosis till death.

Enough.

Abruptly, Emmy stood and walked to the headstone. She kissed her fingers and pressed them against the cold rock.

It's time to go.

She walked back to her car, opened the door, and swung into the driver's seat. After navigating her way out of the cemetery, she headed up to the peninsula ridgeline to the campus of Skyline College.

Much had changed over the years, but she could still drive up to the ridgeline lookout point. As she passed the athletic fields, she couldn't help but glance over at the 3-Day area. She pulled into a parking space. Walking up to the low wall, she sat down and looked out over Pacifica.

She pictured herself sitting here, so long ago, wearing running shorts and a tee shirt, watching that monstrous bank of fog moving relentlessly toward her. Facing her own cowardice in Amy's death was the hardest thing that she had ever had to do, but ultimately, confronting her failure had brought her whole life into focus.

Whenever Emmy thought she might lose that feeling, she'd drive up here and sit in the wind. She'd watch the fog and feel that despair as surely as if she was living in the moment. It was important never to lose it—that emptiness, that hollowness and aching—of losing someone you love. She felt it now, as deeply as she had that day in July of 2001.

It was time to go back home, but she carried the mood with her. She knew she'd have to find her way out of it, but for now, it actually felt good. Sometimes she needed to feel that special hurt.

She got onto the interstate and shot quickly back into town. When she emerged onto the Embarcadero, she went past AT&T Park (Pac Bell Park of the past) and the Embarcadero Center, then turned onto Washington Street. She drove past the Transamerica Pyramid and edged her way into Chinatown. She followed the cable car tracks to Jackson Street, then up the hill to their home.

Reaching up to the visor, she clicked the garage door opener and watched as it rolled up along the ceiling. After parking, she headed up the hallway past the office and studio to the wrought iron spiral stairway that led upstairs to the living quarters.

It was an old house, but roomy, and Emmy loved it dearly. It had been in a Chinese family for many years and Kat had recommended it to them five years ago when they were looking to buy.

It was nearly two-thirty, so she decided to lie down and read before the kids got home from school. She found her book and went into the bedroom. Tossing it on the bed, she sat down at her vanity. As she took off her ear rings, she stared into the mirror.

How much she had changed! Her hair was cut shoulder-length now and parted in the middle. Her face had attained a maturity that was lacking nine years ago. She had managed to keep her weight in line, mostly through walking. She would always be thankful to Barb and Tina for making her do what she herself couldn't.

Glancing up, she looked at the framed photograph of Team Aquatic Park. Standing, she walked over and stood in front of it. She hardly recognized the eighteen year old girl with the puffy eyes, proudly wearing her team baseball cap.

Kat knelt next to her, also looking very, very young.

A great friendship had been born the day they met in the bleachers of Aquatic Park. Hardly a day went by now without them seeing each other. Aunt Kat normally took care of the children after school, along with her own.

Emmy laughed every time she thought about Kat getting married. Her friend had told her so many times that she wanted to marry a Smith or Jones so that people wouldn't sneeze every time she introduced herself, but of course Kat fell in love with Ronnie Chiu, so now *everyone* sneezed when she introduced herself as Kat Chiu. Emmy laughed out loud again just thinking about it.

Dear Kat. Thank God for her.

Her eyes scanned the faces in the picture and fell on Karen and Rhonda. Such a loving mother and daughter. It was a shame that Karen was lost to everyone. That thought brought her eyes to Lauren Sheridan, standing proud, flanked by her guardian angels. So far as Emmy knew, they'd only lost two people in the entire photograph, but she hadn't kept up with everyone.

Next to them were Joy and Ellen. They had gotten married and adopted two beautiful children. They still came to town for some of the group walks and it was always great to see them.

Michael, the gay body builder, stood proud and tall in the back row, his fist raised over his head. He had turned to acting and now had a very successful career. Kat saw him in TV commercials occasionally and said that he was hilarious.

And then there was Janet. Everyone had lost touch with her, but Emmy was still grateful for the wisdom that Janet had passed on to her.

Rachel stood in the third row. They had been friends for quite a while after the Walk, but they'd lost touch a few years back. Maybe it was time to give her old friend a call.

She chuckled when she came to Juliette, her adopted little sister. When the photo had been snapped, Juliette was trying to smile, but she was so cold that it came out as a grimace. She loved Juliette, but the girl hadn't had an easy time of it. There were some women who just had a hard time finding the right man and Juliette definitely fell into that category.

Then there was Tom O'Laughlin. He hadn't changed a bit over the years. Even at fifty-two, he had the same sense of humor and loved his wife to the exclusion of all other women. And when he delivered Josh, the look on his face was amazing. He *was* a damned good doctor and now he was Josh's godfather, as well.

There stood Marianne, with her beautiful smile. When everything fell apart, Marianne kept on walking. It had made Emmy hope that things weren't really falling apart. In fact, it gave everyone a basis to keep walking. Throughout the years, at least once a month, she and

Marianne would test themselves against the hills, often with their friends.

At last, her eyes rested on David Cook.

She'd always assumed that he was the same age as Tom, but, in fact, he had been nearly fifty in 2001. David was the only person she'd ever successfully matched up with anyone, yet from their very first meeting, David and Joanna had hit it off. They dated through summer and into the fall of 2001. He even talked her into doing the 2002 Walk. Everything was going well.

Of course, the 9-11 terrorist attack changed that.

It changed many things.

When the stock markets opened after a three day closure, the Dow fell nearly seven hundred points. David's corporation closed their San Francisco offices in late October. He found it impossible to find work; there were few openings for office managers and hundreds of qualified candidates for each one.

He continued to lead walks into January and February of 2002, but he finally had to capitulate and take a job in Sacramento. Joanna had followed him a few months later. She'd moved into his apartment and that was that. It was by far the best thing Joanna could have done.

But it was devastating for Team Aquatic Park. Marianne and Tom led training walks, but David had been their leader—the glue that held them together. It just wasn't the same without him.

Of course, the hammer hadn't truly fallen yet.

In May of 2002, deep into training for the 3-Day, Avon announced that it was ending its association with Pallotta Teamworks. By the fall, Pallotta was out of business. She remembered David's words to them at O'Reilly's. "I don't begrudge them their income for one minute. They *earn* their fee."

Emmy had been able to raise nearly four thousand dollars for the Walk in 2002, but she walked with the knowledge that this was the last Avon 3-Day Walk. It was something she'd dedicated her life to and it had been rudely pulled out from under her.

Thank goodness the Komen Foundation stepped in. Beginning in November of 2003, Komen picked up the mantle of the 3-Day events. It had been a little rough the first few years, but they kept improving every year. Now, in 2010, Komen was finally poised to exceed the Pallotta/Avon partnership in donations.

Emmy had participated in two San Francisco Komen 3-Day events. The new participants were terribly excited about it and she envied them, but for her everything was different. To begin with, she didn't have the team. In order to maximize her training, she'd led training walks from Aquatic Park and Marianne had joined her, but neither one of them had the nerve to call it Team Aquatic Park. And they didn't walk as a team. And, of course, the route was completely different.

It just wasn't the same.

Emmy sadly shook her head. Here it was, 2010, and they were no closer to finding a cure.

Of course, there were some positive gains. The percentage of women who got breast cancer had fallen to twelve percent. More people discovered breast cancer early and the total number of deaths were down. Those were very good things, but people were still dying every day. Lauren had died. Karen had died.

The real goal had always been to eliminate the damned disease, not just fence it in a little.

She turned her eyes back to David, sitting in the center of the team photo, his white legs glaring when everyone else was bundled up. She smiled. They'd seen each other intermittently over the years and finally he'd landed a job back in the City. The walking club had been revived and they now walked together regularly.

Emmy moved away from the team photo and looked at her wedding picture. May 11, 2002. Ross's hair was neatly trimmed and he looked elegant in his tux. They were married in Pleasanton at the family church. Sarah McMahon had flown up from Los Angeles, Ross's brother was his best man and Grace had been her Maid of Honor.

She slid along the wall to the baby pictures.

Joshua David McMahon. The picture of Josh was taken when he was one year old. Even at that age, Josh had the look of a man. He stared into the lens with confidence, a look of challenge in his green eyes. He seemed very Irish, especially with Ross's little nose and small mouth. His dark brown hair was curly then, but it had smoothed out as he'd grown.

She moved over to look at the photo of her daughter.

Amy Elizabeth McMahon. It had also been taken when she was one year old. Emmy chuckled. Amy was the polar opposite of Josh. In the picture, her face was lit with a huge smile--she'd had the giggles during the photo session. Her hair was bright red then, but it had darkened so that it was now closer to Emmy's color. Her green eyes sparkled with life. Freckles were sprinkled across her nose, just like Emmy. She was a very pretty girl.

Amy was seven years old now and she already wanted to save the world. She was strong and lean--already a first rate walker and a charter member of the new Aquatic Park Walking Club. Amy could take down San Francisco's hills and barely break a sweat. When Emmy had told her about the 3-Day, she'd gone nuts. She wanted to do the Komen walk immediately and when Emmy told her that she'd have to wait eight or nine more years, she'd been grief-stricken.

Emmy's eyes began to fill with tears.

Her day of memory was almost over. Turning, she walked back to their bed, kicked off her shoes, and stretched out. In just a few short minutes, Kat would arrive with Josh and Amy, then there would be homework, dinner and a quiet evening.

If she had learned only one thing in all her years, it was that life is precious, that every breath you take is precious. Amy Fleming might be dead, but she was far from forgotten. Her namesake was a beauty, a real charmer, who would grow up and change the world.

The fire was lit. The torch had been passed.

A new generation would fulfill the promise.

Training Walk Maps

Over the years, as various readers have provided feedback on drafts of this manuscript, I received one comment many times: Please include maps! Heeding that warning, I dove back into my files from 2001 and redesigned the original maps.

If you plan on walking any of these routes for yourself, you will need to keep some things in mind.

The San Francisco of 2001 was a bit different from the San Francisco of today. The obvious example is that Pac Bell Park is currently AT&T Park. Cliff House has been completely remodeled, so the Mechanical Museum is no longer on the lower level and (perhaps sadly, perhaps not so) the hot dog stand is long gone.

The walking maps are rather obviously not to scale. San Francisco has been scrunched in the middle in order to show the whole city west to east and so include the long walks in one picture. The mileage shown is more or less accurate, despite the scrunched map. It looks like a short hike from Lafayette Park to the California Pacific Medical Center, but you'll find it considerably longer.

When the real Team Aquatic Park was training, some of the

walkers were able to cajole the combination to the locked restrooms on the Lobby Level (second floor) of Embarcadero Four. With the fountain, it's a great place to take a break. Otherwise, there should be restrooms at or around every break site.

I've included specific walking directions for each map so if the route seems vague, you can look up the step-by-step directions.

If you really do want to recreate any of these walks, be sure to grab a few partners and a camera, follow David Cook's Safety Instructions, and above all, have fun!

The maps begin on the next page. Originally, the instructions were printed on the back of the maps, but for convenience, I've placed the instructions on the left hand page and the map on the right.

7 Mile Flat Walk

Meet at Aquatic Park

1. Walk east along the Embarcadero, turning south with the street, just past Pier 39. Cross Embarcadero to Embarcadero 4, 2nd Floor (Lobby Level).

BREAK

2. Cross Embarcadero and continue south on Embarcadero to Pac Bell Park. Circle statue of Willie Mays and return to Embarcadero 4.

BREAK

3. Cross Embarcadero and continue north and west to Aquatic Park.

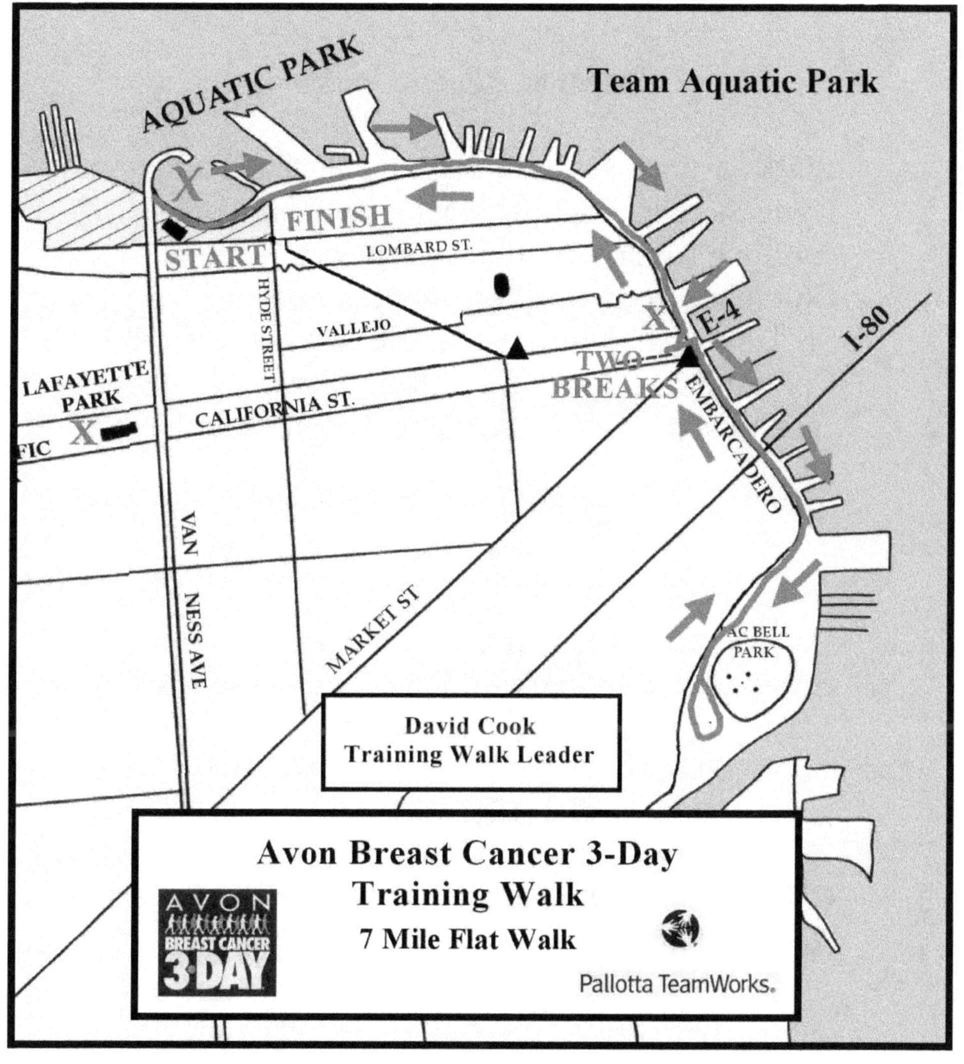

AQUATIC PARK
Team Aquatic Park
FINISH
START
LOMBARD ST.
HYDE STREET
VALLEJO
E-4
I-80
TWO BREAKS
LAFAYETTE PARK
CALIFORNIA ST.
EMBARCADERO
VAN NESS AVE
MARKET ST
PAC BELL PARK
David Cook
Training Walk Leader
Avon Breast Cancer 3-Day
Training Walk
7 Mile Flat Walk
AVON BREAST CANCER 3-DAY
Pallotta TeamWorks.

8 Mile Hill/Flat Walk

Meet at Aquatic Park

1. Walk east and south through Cable Car Turnaround to Hyde St. Head uphill. Meet at Lombard, then continue south to Vallejo. Turn east on Vallejo, cross Columbus, turn north on Grant Ave. and go to Union St. Turn east up hill to summit, just below Coit Tower. Continue east down hill to Levi Plaza, then along Embarcadero to Embarcadero 4, 2nd Floor (Lobby Level).

BREAK

2. Cross Embarcadero and continue south on Embarcadero to Pac Bell Park. Circle statue of Willie Mays and return to Embarcadero 4.

BREAK

3. Cross Embarcadero and continue north and west to Aquatic Park.

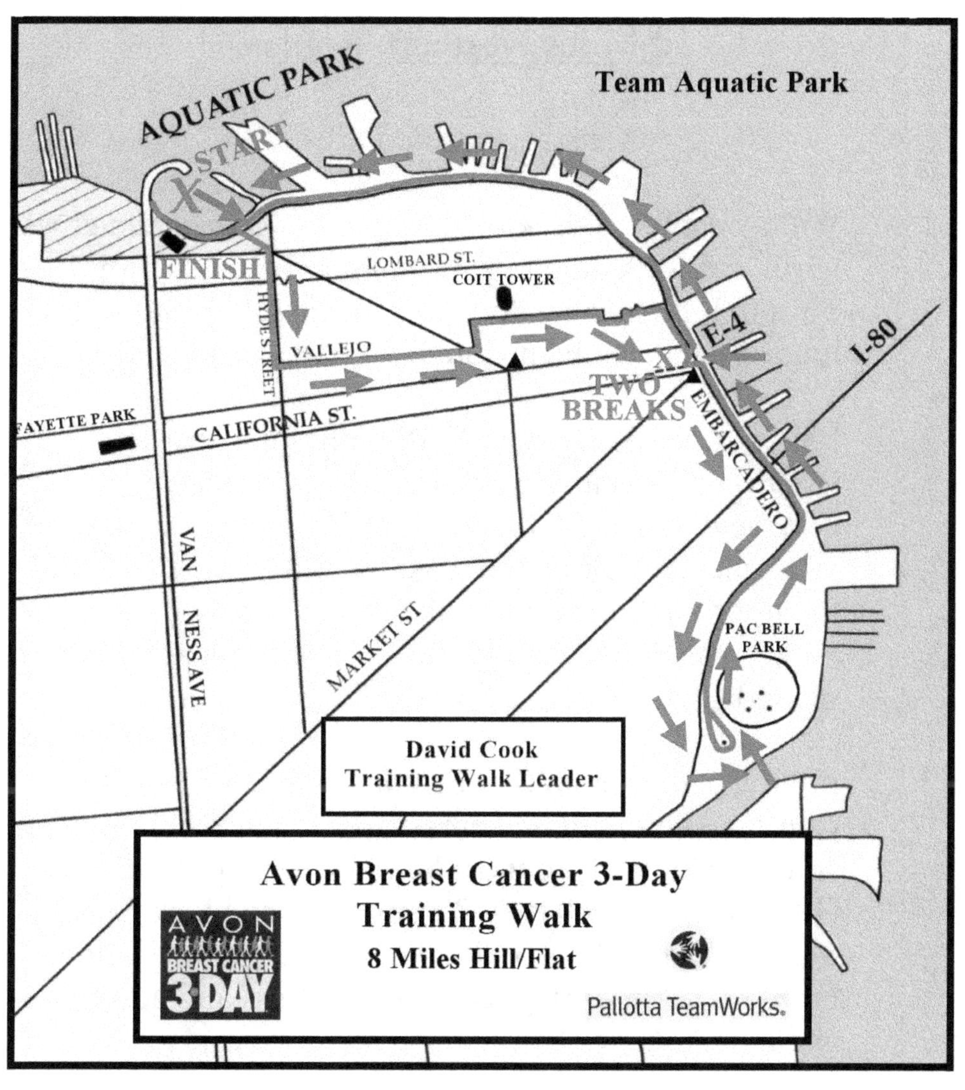
Team Aquatic Park
AQUATIC PARK
START
FINISH
LOMBARD ST.
COIT TOWER
HYDE STREET
VALLEJO
E-4
I-80
TWO
BREAKS
EMBARCADERO
FAYETTE PARK
CALIFORNIA ST.
VAN NESS AVE
MARKET ST
PAC BELL PARK
David Cook
Training Walk Leader
Avon Breast Cancer 3-Day
Training Walk
8 Miles Hill/Flat
AVON
BREAST CANCER
3-DAY
Pallotta TeamWorks.

10 Miles Northern Route

Meet at Aquatic Park

1. Walk west through Fort Mason and Marina, then cross north and walk along the beach nearly to Fort Point. Turn uphill on Long Ave. to Lincoln Blvd. and follow it north to the Golden Gate Bridge Plaza and BREAK.

2. Follow Lincoln Blvd. to Fort Scott, then veer left (south) on Washington and follow it to Battery Caulfield. Go south on BC until it becomes Wedemeyer. Follow that past the old Marine Hospital to out of the Presidio to Lake Ave. Turning east, cross Park Presidio and turn left to Mountain Lake for the second BREAK.

3. Follow path east up past driving range to Arguello. Continue downhill and cross over to Pacific Ave. at Julius Kahn Playground. Continue east up Pacific St. Hill and on to Pierce St. Turn north one block to Vallejo, then follow Vallejo east to Franklin. Follow Franklin north to Bay, Bay to Van Ness and north again to Aquatic Park.

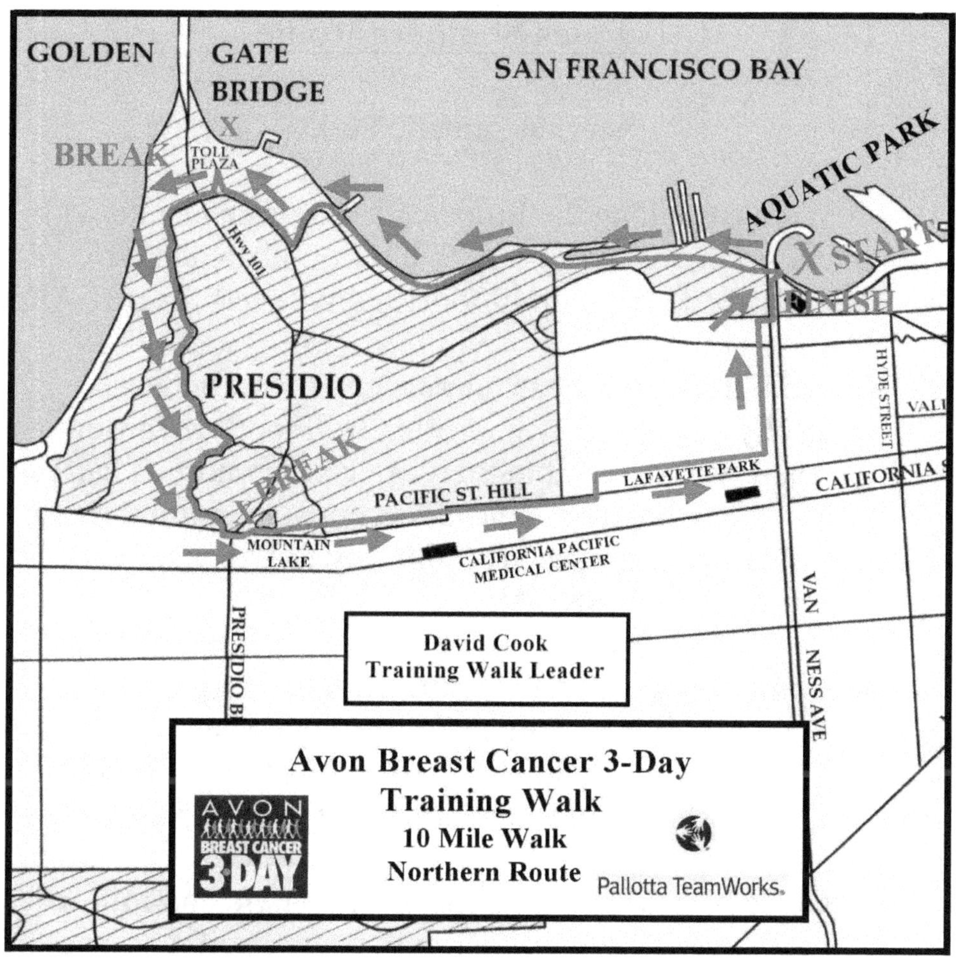
GOLDEN GATE BRIDGE
SAN FRANCISCO BAY
BREAK
TOLL PLAZA
Hwy 101
AQUATIC PARK
START
FINISH
PRESIDIO
BREAK
HYDE STREET
PACIFIC ST. HILL
LAFAYETTE PARK
CALIFORNIA
MOUNTAIN LAKE
CALIFORNIA PACIFIC MEDICAL CENTER
VAN NESS AVE
PRESIDIO B
David Cook
Training Walk Leader
Avon Breast Cancer 3-Day
Training Walk
10 Mile Walk
Northern Route
AVON BREAST CANCER 3-DAY
Pallotta TeamWorks.

10 Miles Southern Route

Meet at Aquatic Park

1. Walk east along the Embarcadero, turning south with the street, just past Pier 39. Cross Embarcadero to Embarcadero 4, 2nd Floor (Lobby Level) for BREAK.

2. Walk through Embarcadero Center west between Lobby Level and Promenade (3rd Floor) to Sansome where you descend to Street Level. Jag north a half block to Clay St. and head west up a long hill through Chinatown. Continue all the way to Lafayette Park for the second BREAK.

3. Come south out of Lafayette Park to Sacramento. Follow it west to Spruce St., then jag south to California and follow it up the block to the California Pacific Medical Center for the third BREAK.

4. Go east back up California to Spruce St. and follow it north over a little hill. Drop down to Pacific St. and turn east up the Pacific St. hill. Continue to Pierce St. Turn north one block to Vallejo, then follow Vallejo east to Franklin. Follow Franklin north to Bay, Bay to Van Ness and north again to Aquatic Park.

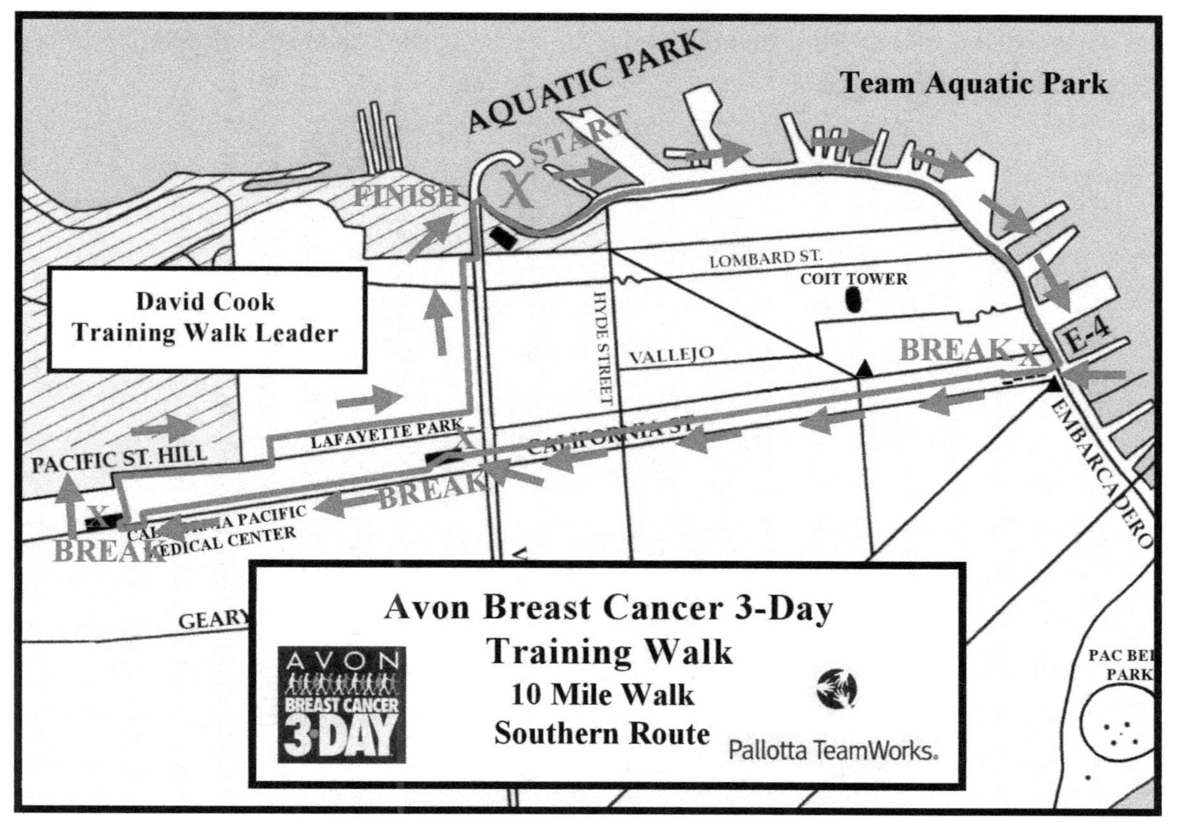
AQUATIC PARK
Team Aquatic Park
START
FINISH
LOMBARD ST.
COIT TOWER
HYDE STREET
VALLEJO
BREAK
E-4
EMBARCADERO
LAFAYETTE PARK
CALIFORNIA ST.
PACIFIC ST. HILL
BREAK
BREAK
MEDICAL CENTER
GEARY
PAC BE
PARK
David Cook
Training Walk Leader
Avon Breast Cancer 3-Day
Training Walk
10 Mile Walk
Southern Route
AVON
BREAST CANCER
3-DAY
Pallotta TeamWorks.

10 Mile Flat Walk

Meet at Aquatic Park

1. Walk east along the Embarcadero, turning south with the street, just past Pier 39. Cross Embarcadero to Embarcadero 4, 2nd Floor (Lobby Level) for BREAK.

2. Cross Embarcadero and continue south on Embarcadero to Pac Bell Park. Circle statue of Willie Mays and return to Embarcadero 4 for second BREAK.

3. Cross Embarcadero and continue north and west to Aquatic Park for a third BREAK.

4. Continue west through Fort Mason and down to Marina Blvd. Follow it to Baker St. and turn south past the Palace of Fine Arts. At Chestnut St. cross Richardson and continue east past Moscone Rec. Center, then turn north on Laguna. Follow it to Bay St. and turn east to Van Ness and north to Aquatic Park.

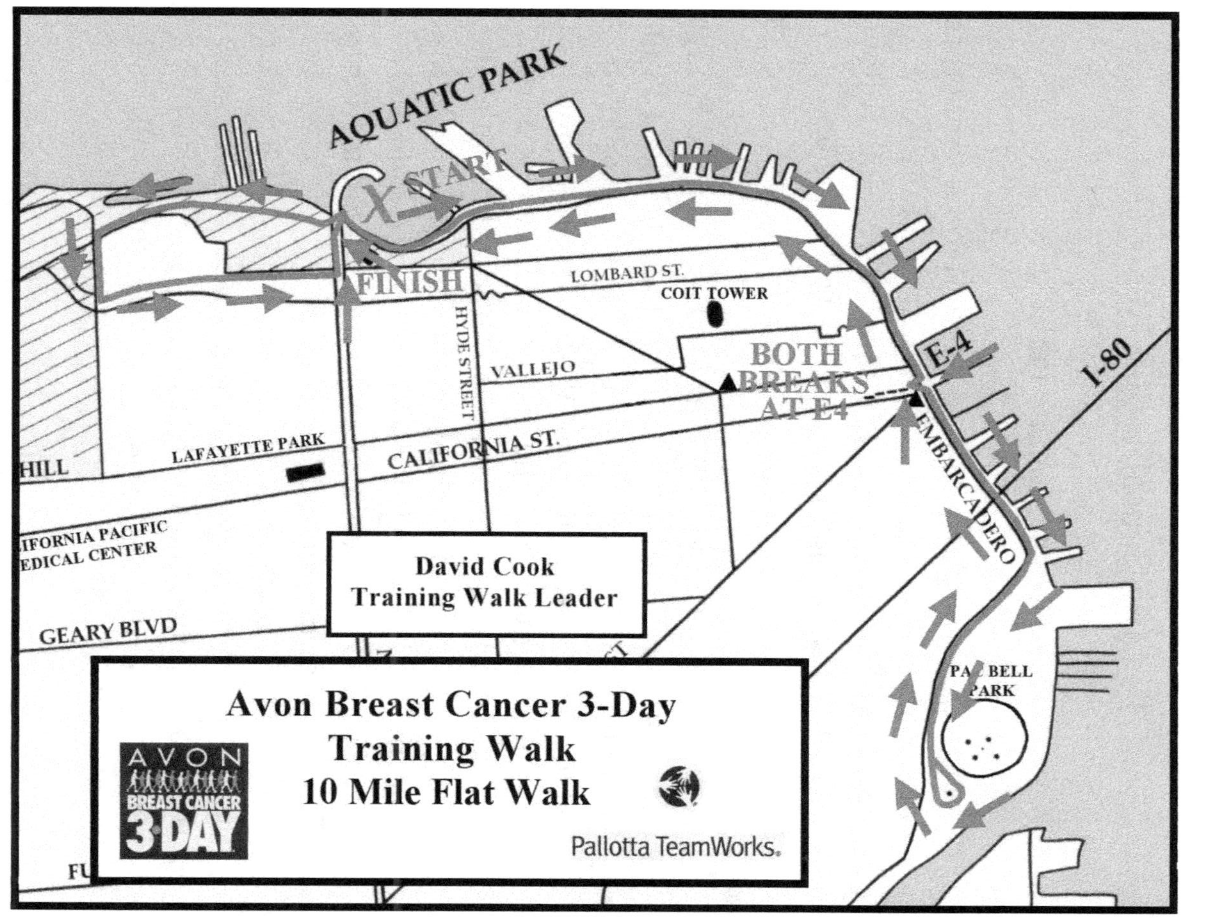
AQUATIC PARK
START
FINISH
LOMBARD ST.
COIT TOWER
HYDE STREET
VALLEJO
BOTH BREAKS AT E4
E-4
I-80
EMBARCADERO
LAFAYETTE PARK
CALIFORNIA ST.
HILL
GEARY BLVD
David Cook
Training Walk Leader
Avon Breast Cancer 3-Day
Training Walk
10 Mile Flat Walk
AVON BREAST CANCER 3-DAY
Pallotta TeamWorks

10 Mile Sausalito Fun Walk

Meet at Aquatic Park

1. Walk west through Fort Mason and Marina, then cross north and walk along the beach nearly to Fort Point. Turn uphill on Long Ave. to Lincoln Blvd. and follow it north to the Golden Gate Bridge Toll Plaza and BREAK.

2. Continue up through Toll Plaza to Golden Gate Bridge and walk north across it. Continue past the Vista Point until you reach Alexander Ave. Follow it east down the hill all the way into Sausalito. It becomes South St. then turns right to become 2nd St. Follow that north until Richardson. Turn right and follow it down to the shore. It will veer left and become Bridgeway. Follow it north to Viña del Mar Park. Turn to the right and you will find yourself at Sausalito Point and the Ferry Terminal for the second BREAK.

3. If you return by ferry, disembark at Pier 39 and walk west to Aquatic Park for 10 miles. If you return by walking back the way you came, your total walk will be about 18.5 miles.

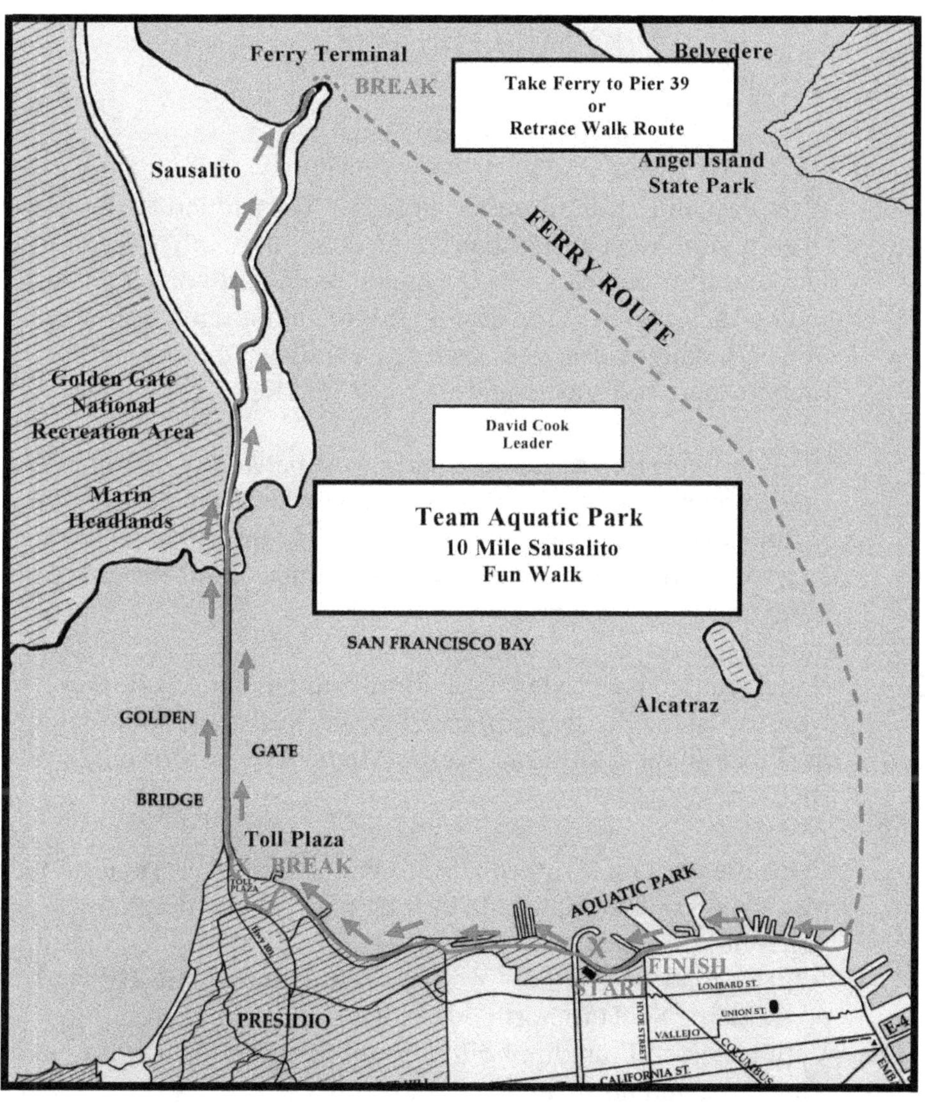

Ferry Terminal
BREAK
Belvedere
Take Ferry to Pier 39
or
Retrace Walk Route
Sausalito
Angel Island
State Park
FERRY ROUTE
Golden Gate
National
Recreation Area
David Cook
Leader
Marin
Headlands
Team Aquatic Park
10 Mile Sausalito
Fun Walk
SAN FRANCISCO BAY
Alcatraz
GOLDEN
GATE
BRIDGE
Toll Plaza
BREAK
AQUATIC PARK
FINISH
START
LOMBARD ST.
UNION ST.
HYDE STREET
VALLEJO
COLUMBUS
PRESIDIO
CALIFORNIA ST.
E-4

12 Mile Hill Walk

Meet at Aquatic Park

1. Walk east and south through Cable Car Turnaround to Hyde St. Head uphill. Meet at Lombard, then continue south to Vallejo. Turn east on Vallejo, cross Columbus, turn north on Grant Ave. and go to Union St. Turn east up hill to summit, just below Coit Tower. Continue east down hill to Levi Plaza, then along Embarcadero to Embarcadero 4 for BREAK.

2. Walk through Embarcadero Center west between Lobby Level and Promenade (3rd Floor) to Sansome where you descend to Street Level. Jag north a half block to Clay St. and head west up a long hill through Chinatown. Continue all the way to Lafayette Park for the second BREAK.

3. Come south out of Lafayette Park to Sacramento. Follow it west to Spruce St., then jag south to California and follow it up the block to the California Pacific Medical Center for the third BREAK.

4. Continue west on California St. to Park Presidio. Turn north to Mountain Lake. Follow path east up past driving range to Arguello. Continue downhill and cross over to Pacific Ave. at Julius Kahn Playground. Continue east up Pacific St. Hill and on to Pierce St. Turn north one block to Vallejo, then follow Vallejo east to Franklin. Follow Franklin north to Bay, Bay to Van Ness, and north again to Aquatic Park.

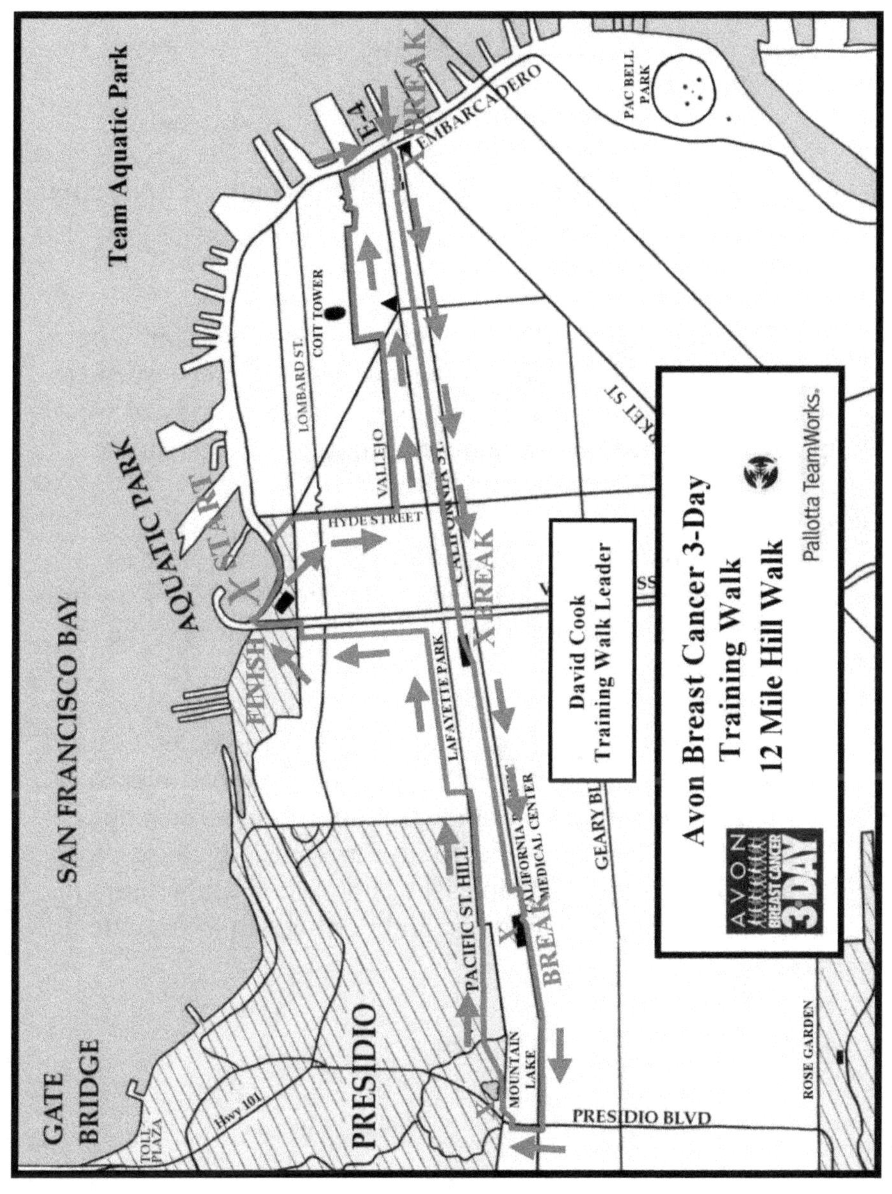
Team Aquatic Park
SAN FRANCISCO BAY
AQUATIC PARK
GATE
BRIDGE
TOLL PLAZA
Hwy 101
PRESIDIO
MOUNTAIN LAKE
PRESIDIO BLVD
PACIFIC ST. HILL
LAFAYETTE PARK
MEDICAL CENTER
HYDE STREET
VALLEJO
LOMBARD ST.
COIT TOWER
EMBARCADERO
PAC BELL PARK
ROSE GARDEN
START
FINISH
BREAK
BREAK
BREAK
E-4
David Cook
Training Walk Leader
Avon Breast Cancer 3-Day
Training Walk
12 Mile Hill Walk
AVON
BREAST CANCER
3-DAY
Pallotta TeamWorks.

13 Mile Walk

Meet at Aquatic Park

1. Walk east along the Embarcadero, turning south with the street, just past Pier 39. Cross Embarcadero to Embarcadero 4, 2nd Floor (Lobby Level) for BREAK.

2. Walk through Embarcadero Center west between Lobby Level and Promenade (3rd Floor) to Sansome where you descend to Street Level. Jag north a half block to Clay St. and head west up a long hill through Chinatown. Continue all the way to Lafayette Park for the second BREAK.

3. Come south out of Lafayette Park to Sacramento. Follow it west to Spruce St., then jag south to California and follow it up the block to the California Pacific Medical Center for the third BREAK.

4. Continue west to Arguello and turn north until you enter the Presidio. Turn right on the path downhill and cross over to Pacific Ave. at Julius Kahn Playground. Continue east up Pacific St. Hill and on to Pierce St. Turn north one block to Vallejo, then follow Vallejo east to Franklin. Follow Franklin north to Bay, Bay to Van Ness, and north again to Aquatic Park.

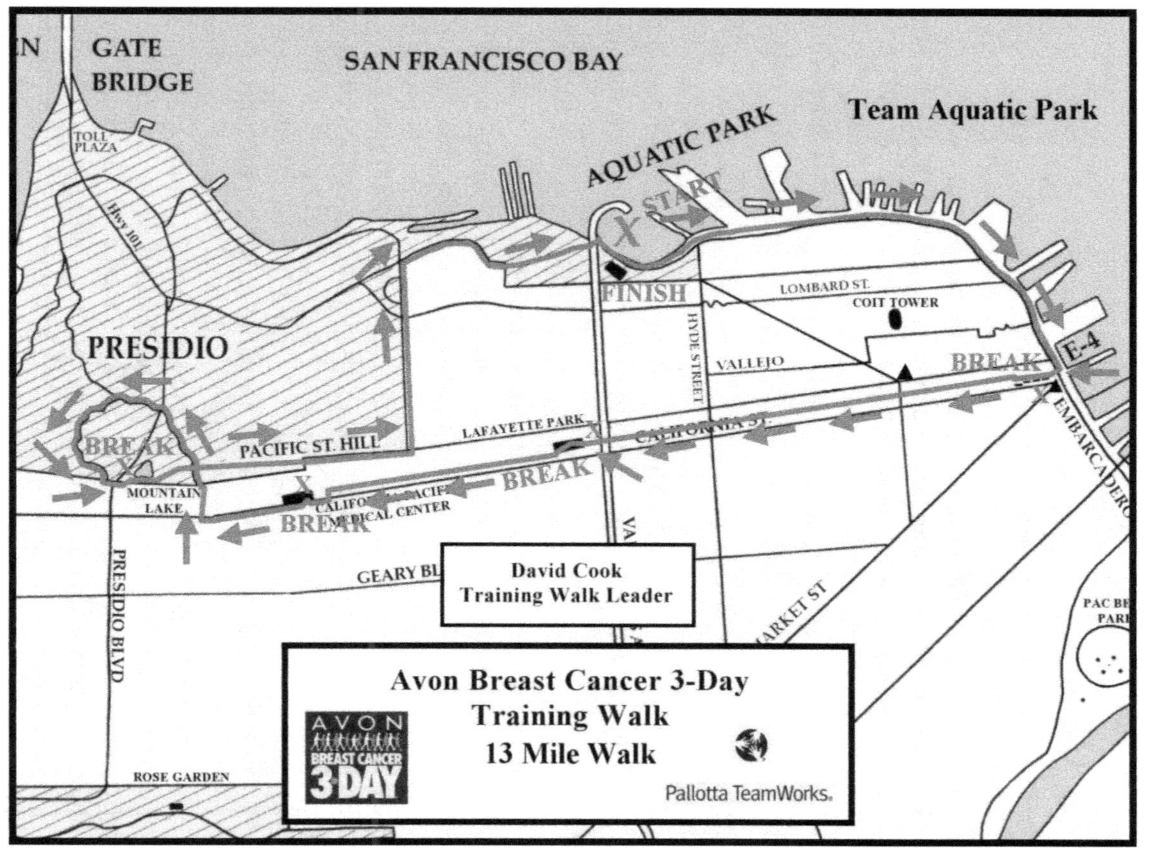

GATE BRIDGE
SAN FRANCISCO BAY
Team Aquatic Park
AQUATIC PARK
TOLL PLAZA
Hwy 101
START
FINISH
LOMBARD ST.
COIT TOWER
PRESIDIO
HYDE STREET
VALLEJO
BREAK
E-4
LAFAYETTE PARK
CALIFORNIA ST.
PACIFIC ST. HILL
BREAK
BREAK
MOUNTAIN LAKE
CALIFO MEDICAL CENTER
BREAK
EMBARCADERO
GEARY BL
David Cook
Training Walk Leader
MARKET ST
PRESIDIO BLVD
Avon Breast Cancer 3-Day
Training Walk
13 Mile Walk
AVON BREAST CANCER 3-DAY
ROSE GARDEN
Pallotta TeamWorks.

14 Mile Hill Walk

Meet at Aquatic Park

1. Walk east and south through Cable Car Turnaround to Hyde St. Head uphill. Meet at Lombard, then continue south to Vallejo. Turn east on Vallejo, cross Columbus, turn north on Grant Ave. and go to Union St. Turn east up hill to summit, just below Coit Tower. Continue east down hill to Levi Plaza, then along Embarcadero to Embarcadero 4 for BREAK.

2. Walk through Embarcadero Center west between Lobby Level and Promenade (3rd Floor) to Sansome where you descend to Street Level. Jag north a half block to Clay St. and head west up a long hill through Chinatown. Continue all the way to Lafayette Park for the second BREAK.

3. Come south out of Lafayette Park to Sacramento. Follow it west to Spruce St., then jag south to California and follow it up the block to the California Pacific Medical Center for the third BREAK.

4. Continue west on California St. to Arguello. Turn north into the Presidio. Continuing north past the golf course, follow the path left roughly following Arguello. You come out on Washington. Follow it to Battery Caulfield. Go south on BC until it becomes Wedemeyer. Follow that past the old Marine Hospital to out of the Presidio to Lake Ave. Turning east, cross Park Presidio and turn left to Mountain Lake. Follow path east up past driving range to Arguello. Continue downhill and cross over to Pacific Ave. at Julius Kahn Playground. Continue east up Pacific St. Hill and on to Pierce St. Turn north one block to Vallejo, then follow Vallejo east to Franklin. Follow Franklin north to Bay, Bay to Van Ness and north again to Aquatic Park.

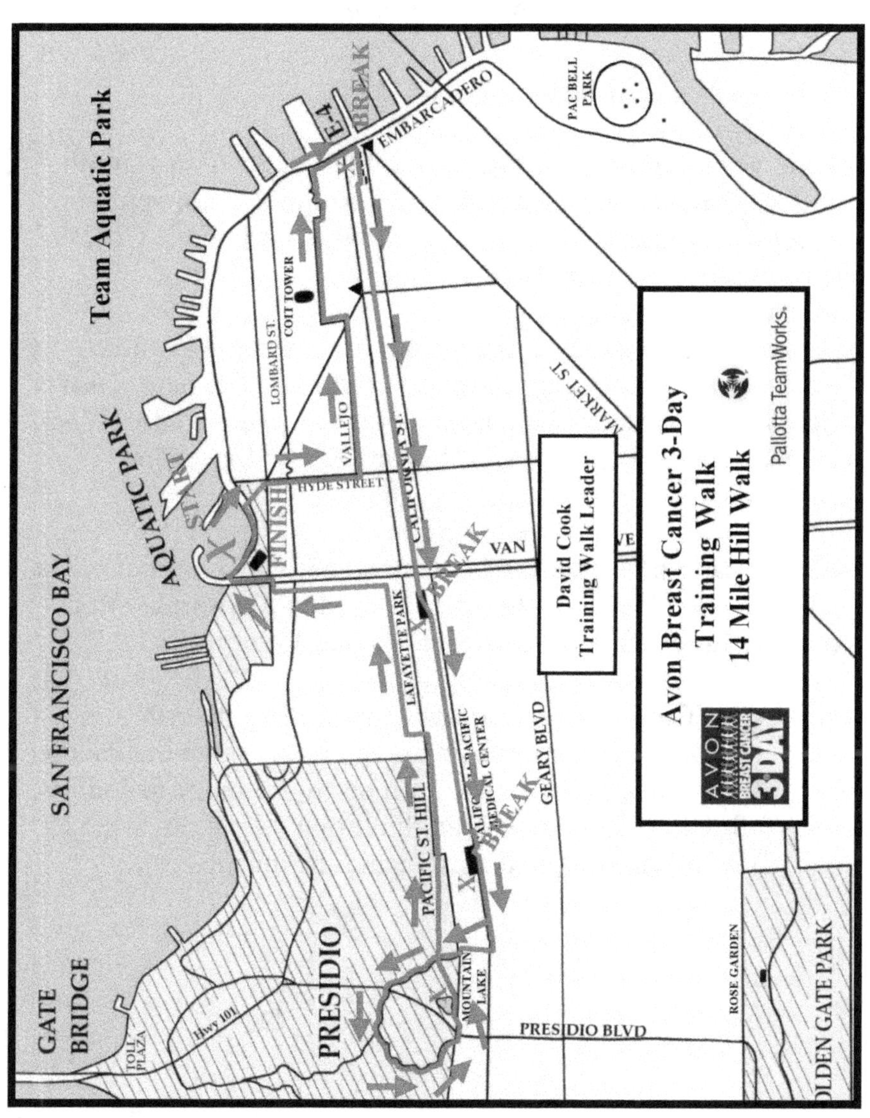
Team Aquatic Park
SAN FRANCISCO BAY
AQUATIC PARK
GATE BRIDGE
TOLL PLAZA
Hwy 101
PRESIDIO
MOUNTAIN LAKE
PACIFIC ST. HILL
MEDICAL CENTER
BREAK
GEARY BLVD
PRESIDIO BLVD
ROSE GARDEN
OLDEN GATE PARK
LAFAYETTE PARK
FINISH
START
HYDE STREET
VALLEJO
LOMBARD ST.
COIT TOWER
CALIFORNIA ST.
VAN
MARKET ST
E-4
EMBARCADERO
PAC BELL PARK
David Cook
Training Walk Leader
Avon Breast Cancer 3-Day
Training Walk
14 Mile Hill Walk
AVON BREAST CANCER 3-DAY
Pallotta TeamWorks.

14.5 Mile Walk

Meet at Aquatic Park

1. Walk west through Fort Mason and Marina, then cross north and walk along the beach nearly to Fort Point. Turn uphill on Long Ave. to Lincoln Blvd. and follow it north to the Golden Gate Bridge Plaza and BREAK.

2. Follow Lincoln Blvd. all the way until it exits the Presidio. Veer right to 25th Ave. and follow it south to Clement. Turn right and go west on Clement to 40th Ave. Turn south a block to Geary Blvd. Follow it west to Cliff House for second BREAK.

3. Follow path in reverse to Clement and 25th Ave. Turn north at 25th for one block to California St. Follow California Street east to California Pacific Medical Center for third BREAK.

4. Go east up California to Spruce St. and follow it north over a little hill. Drop down to Pacific St. and turn east up the Pacific St. hill. Continue to Pierce St. Turn north one block to Vallejo, then follow Vallejo east to Franklin. Follow Franklin north to Bay, Bay to Van Ness and north again to Aquatic Park.

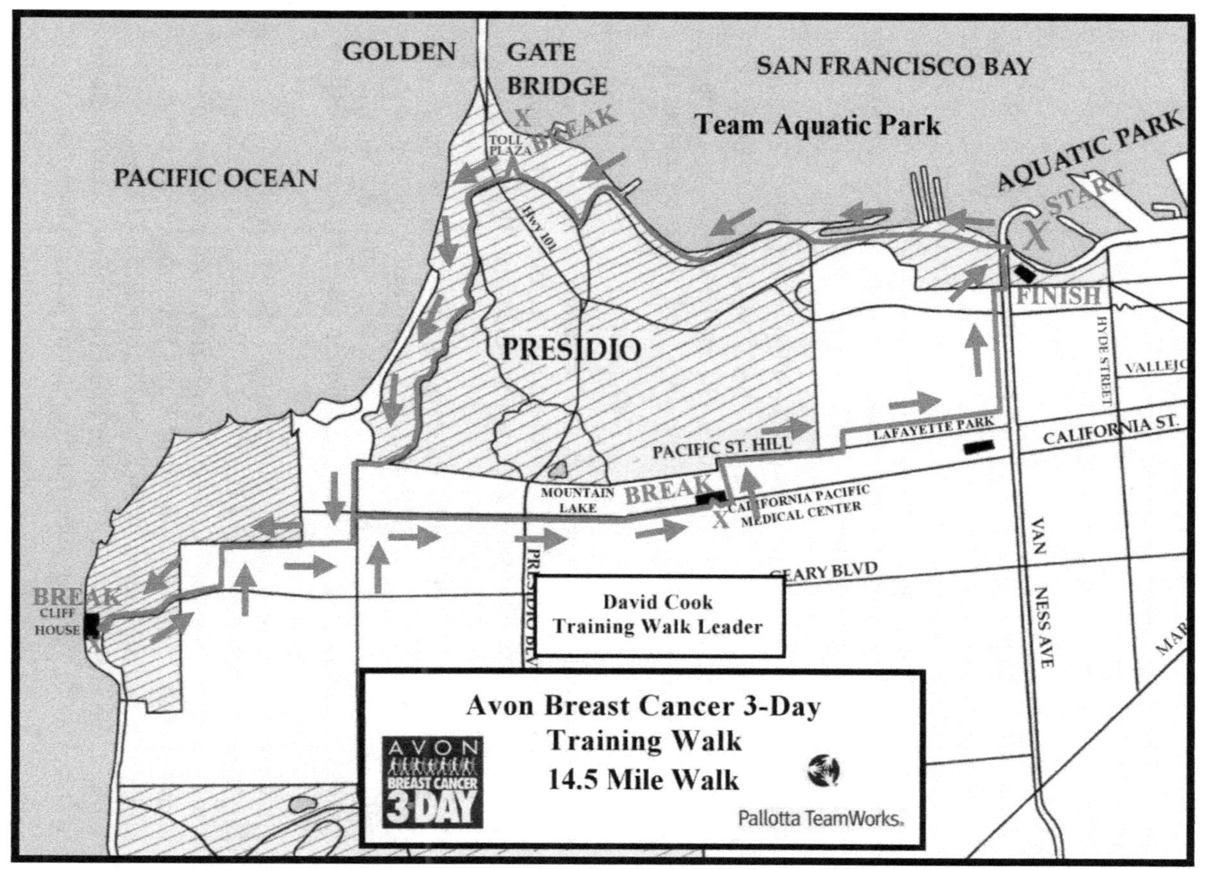
GOLDEN
GATE
BRIDGE
SAN FRANCISCO BAY
Team Aquatic Park
BREAK
TOLL PLAZA
PACIFIC OCEAN
Hwy 101
AQUATIC PARK
START
FINISH
PRESIDIO
HYDE STREET
VALLEJO
LAFAYETTE PARK
CALIFORNIA ST.
PACIFIC ST. HILL
MOUNTAIN LAKE
BREAK
CALIFORNIA PACIFIC MEDICAL CENTER
VAN NESS AVE
PRESIDIO BLVD
GEARY BLVD
BREAK
CLIFF HOUSE
David Cook
Training Walk Leader
Avon Breast Cancer 3-Day
Training Walk
14.5 Mile Walk
AVON BREAST CANCER 3-DAY
Pallotta TeamWorks

15 Mile Hill Walk

Meet at Aquatic Park

1. Walk east and south through Cable Car Turnaround to Hyde St. Head uphill. Meet at Lombard, then continue south to Vallejo. Turn east on Vallejo, cross Columbus, turn north on Grant Ave. and go to Union St. Turn east up hill to summit, just below Coit Tower. Continue east down hill to Levi Plaza, then along Embarcadero to Embarcadero 4 for BREAK.

2. Walk through Embarcadero Center west between Lobby Level and Promenade (3rd Floor) to Sansome where you descend to Street Level. Jag north a half block to Clay St. and head west up a long hill through Chinatown. Continue all the way to Lafayette Park for the second BREAK.

3. Come south out of Lafayette Park to Sacramento. Follow it west to Spruce St., then jag south to California and follow it up the block to the California Pacific Medical Center for the third BREAK.

4. Follow Commonwealth south to Geary and cross onto Stanyan. Follow Stanyan south to Golden Gate Park. Cross Fulton St. and walk along the park to Park Presidio, then turn north and walk to Lake Ave. Cross Park Presidio to Mountain Lake for fourth BREAK.

5. Go west on Lake to enter the Presidio on 14th Ave. Follow Wedemeyer north to Battery Caulfield to Washington and loop around the Presidio Golf Course to Arguello. Turn east and downhill. Cross over to Pacific Ave. at Julius Kahn Playground. Continue east up Pacific St. Hill and on to Pierce St. Turn north one block to Vallejo, then follow Vallejo east to Franklin. Follow Franklin north to Bay, Bay to Van Ness and north again to Aquatic Park.

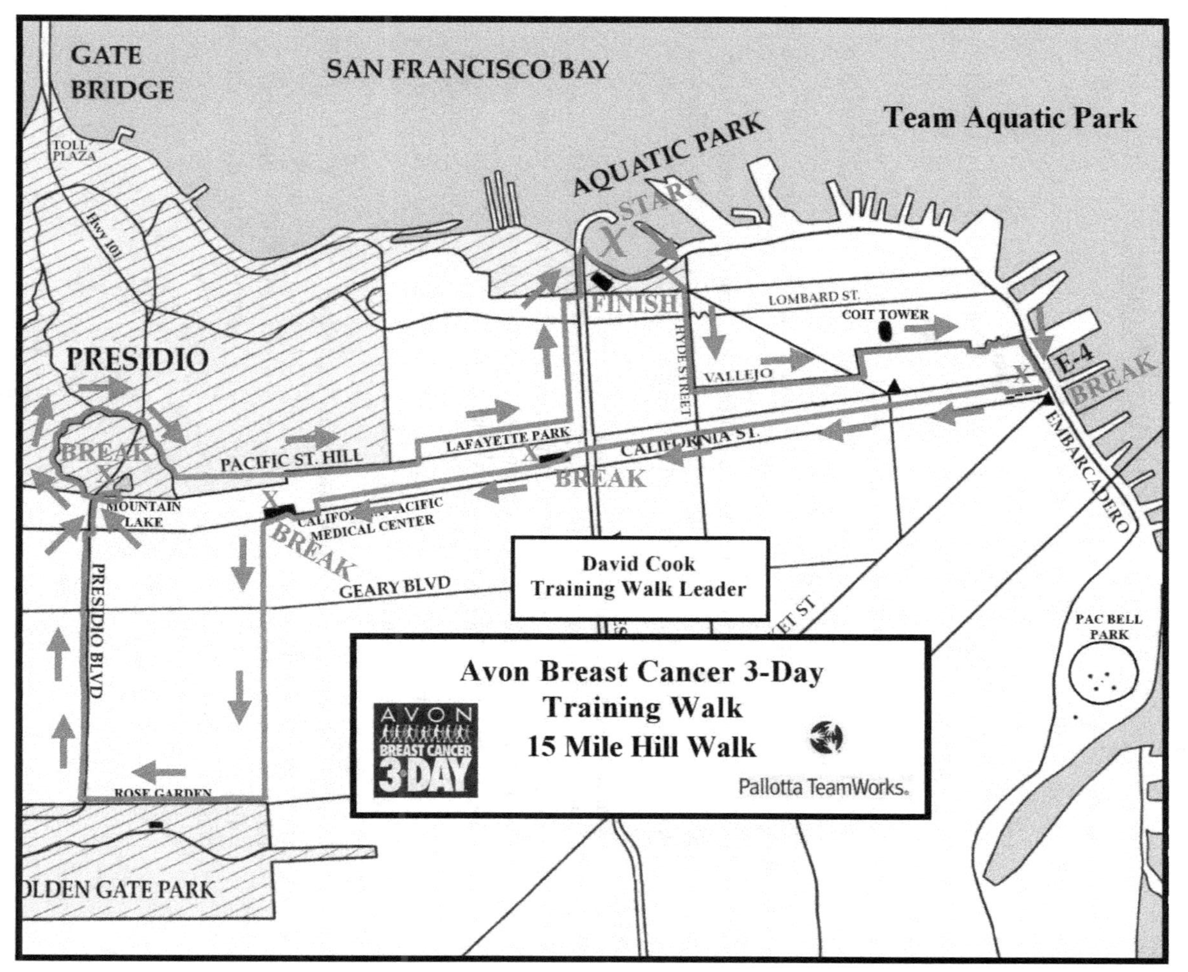
GATE
BRIDGE
SAN FRANCISCO BAY
Team Aquatic Park
TOLL PLAZA
Hwy 101
AQUATIC PARK
START
FINISH
LOMBARD ST.
COIT TOWER
HYDE STREET
VALLEJO
E-4
BREAK
PRESIDIO
BREAK
MOUNTAIN LAKE
PACIFIC ST. HILL
LAFAYETTE PARK
CALIFORNIA ST.
BREAK
MEDICAL CENTER
BREAK
EMBARCADERO
GEARY BLVD
David Cook
Training Walk Leader
PRESIDIO BLVD
PAC BELL PARK
Avon Breast Cancer 3-Day
Training Walk
15 Mile Hill Walk
AVON BREAST CANCER 3-DAY
Pallotta TeamWorks.
ROSE GARDEN
OLDEN GATE PARK

15 Miles - Southern Route

Meet at Aquatic Park

1. Walk east along the Embarcadero, turning south with the street, just past Pier 39. Cross Embarcadero to Embarcadero 4, 2nd Floor (Lobby Level) for BREAK.

2. Walk through Embarcadero Center west between Lobby Level and Promenade (3rd Floor) to Sansome where you descend to Street Level. Jag north a half block to Clay St. and head west up a long hill through Chinatown. Continue all the way to Lafayette Park for the second BREAK.

3. Come south out of Lafayette Park to Sacramento. Follow it west to Spruce St., then jag south to California and follow it up the block to the California Pacific Medical Center for the third BREAK.

4. Continue west to Arguello and turn north until you enter the Presidio. Continuing north past the golf course, follow the path left roughly following Arguello. You come out on Washington. Follow it to Battery Caulfield. Go south on BC until it becomes Wedemeyer. Follow that past the old Marine Hospital to out of the Presidio to California St. Turn west to 18th Ave. Follow 18th Ave. south to Fulton. Walk along the park to Park Presidio, then turn north and follow it to Lake St. Turning east, cross Park Presidio and turn left to Mountain Lake for the fourth BREAK.

5. Follow path east up past driving range to Arguello. Continue downhill and cross over to Pacific Ave. at Julius Kahn Playground. Continue east up Pacific St. Hill and on to Pierce St. Turn north one block to Vallejo, then follow Vallejo east to Franklin. Follow Franklin north to Bay, Bay to Van Ness and north again to Aquatic Park.

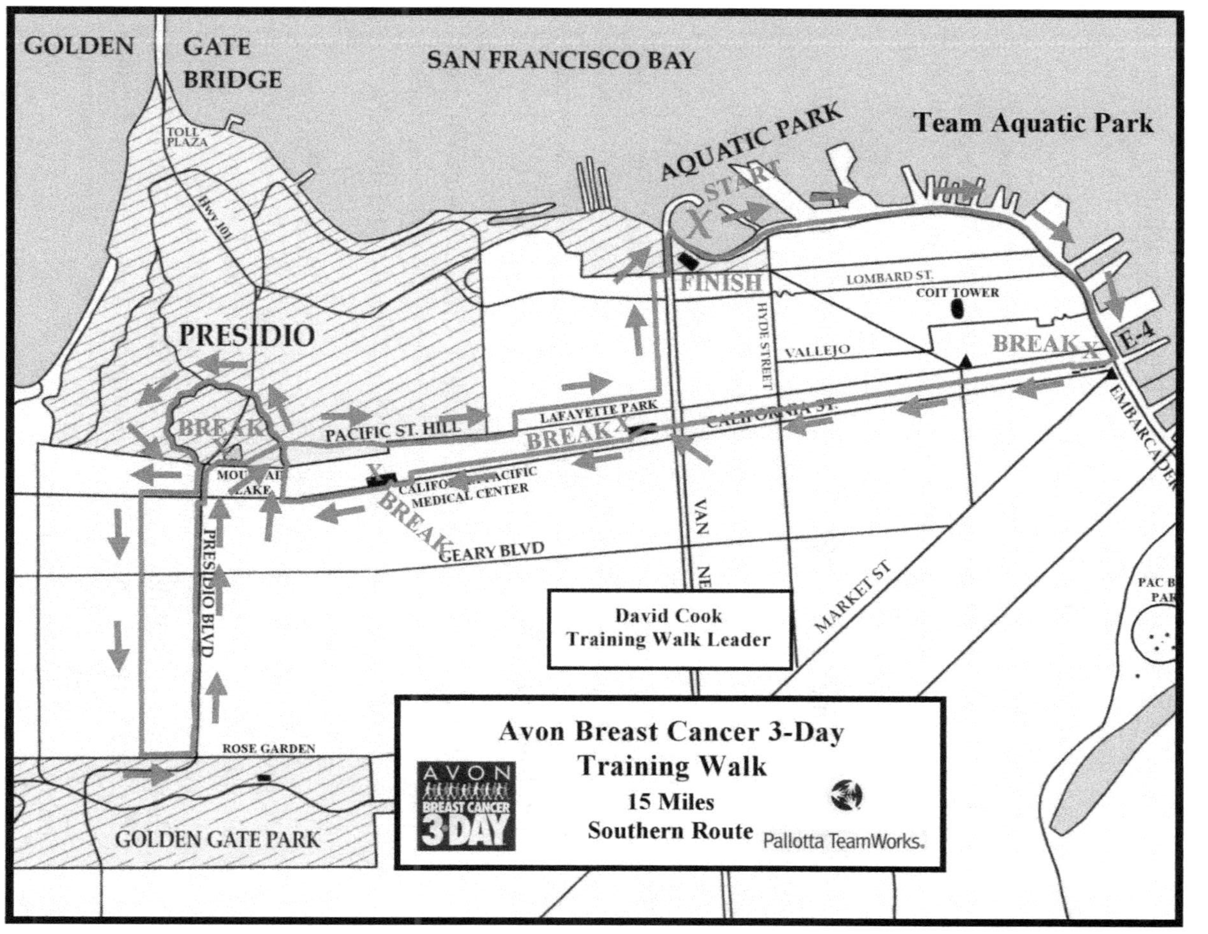

GOLDEN GATE BRIDGE
SAN FRANCISCO BAY
Team Aquatic Park
AQUATIC PARK
START
FINISH
TOLL PLAZA
Hwy 101
PRESIDIO
BREAK
PACIFIC ST. HILL
LAFAYETTE PARK
CALIFORNIA ST.
LOMBARD ST.
COIT TOWER
VALLEJO
HYDE STREET
E-4
EMBARCADERO
MEDICAL CENTER
GEARY BLVD
VAN NESS
MARKET ST
PRESIDIO BLVD
ROSE GARDEN
GOLDEN GATE PARK
David Cook
Training Walk Leader
Avon Breast Cancer 3-Day
Training Walk
15 Miles
Southern Route
AVON BREAST CANCER 3-DAY
Pallotta TeamWorks.

15 Mile Walk - Northern Route

Meet at Aquatic Park

1. Walk west through Fort Mason and Marina, then cross north and walk along the beach nearly to Fort Point. Turn uphill on Long Ave. to Lincoln Blvd. and follow it north to the Golden Gate Bridge Plaza and BREAK.

2. Follow Lincoln Blvd. all the way to the Baker Beach road. Turn right on it and follow down to the beach for second BREAK.

3. Return to Lincoln and follow until it exits the Presidio. Veer right to 25th Ave. and follow it south to Clement. Turn right and go west on Clement to 36th Ave. Turn south and walk to Fulton, then cross into Golden Gate Park on John F. Kennedy and follow it east to Sprekel's Lake for third BREAK.

3\. Follow JFK to the Asian Art Museum, then turn north and get onto Park Presidio. Walk north to Lake St. Cross over Park Presidio east and go to Mountain Lake for fourth BREAK.

4\. Go west on Lake to enter the Presidio on 14th Ave. Follow Wedemeyer north to Battery Caulfield to Washington and loop around the Presidio Golf Course to Arguello. Turn east and downhill. Cross over to Pacific Ave. at Julius Kahn Playground. Continue east up Pacific St. Hill and on to Pierce St. Turn north one block to Vallejo, then follow Vallejo east to Franklin. Follow Franklin north to Bay, Bay to Van Ness and north again to Aquatic Park.

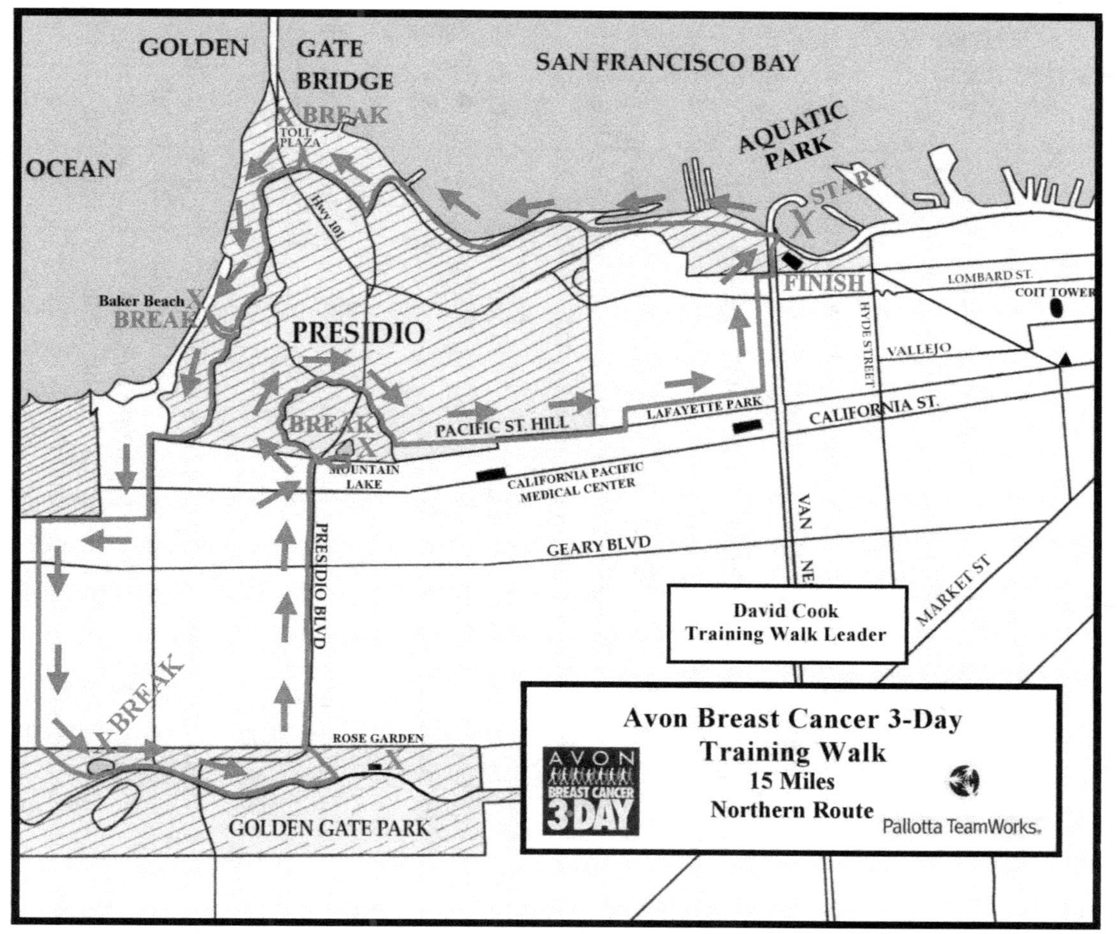
GOLDEN
GATE
BRIDGE
SAN FRANCISCO BAY
AQUATIC PARK
START
FINISH
BREAK
TOLL PLAZA
OCEAN
Hwy 101
Baker Beach
BREAK
PRESIDIO
BREAK
MOUNTAIN LAKE
PACIFIC ST. HILL
LAFAYETTE PARK
CALIFORNIA ST.
CALIFORNIA PACIFIC MEDICAL CENTER
LOMBARD ST.
COIT TOWER
HYDE STREET
VALLEJO
VAN NESS
GEARY BLVD
PRESIDIO BLVD
MARKET ST
BREAK
ROSE GARDEN
GOLDEN GATE PARK
David Cook
Training Walk Leader
Avon Breast Cancer 3-Day
Training Walk
15 Miles
Northern Route
AVON BREAST CANCER 3-DAY
Pallotta TeamWorks.

16 Mile Walk - Day 2 Sim

Meet at Aquatic Park

1. Walk east along the Embarcadero, turning south with the street, just past Pier 39. Cross Embarcadero to Embarcadero 4, 2nd Floor (Lobby Level) for BREAK.

2. Walk through Embarcadero Center west between Lobby Level and Promenade (3rd Floor) to Sansome where you descend to Street Level. Jag north a half block to Clay St. and head west up a long hill through Chinatown. Continue all the way to Lafayette Park for the second BREAK.

3. Come south out of Lafayette Park to Sacramento. Follow it west to Spruce St., then jag south to California and follow it up the block to the California Pacific Medical Center for the third BREAK.

4. Continue west on California to 25th Ave. Turn south and continue into Golden Gate Park, going east on John F. Kennedy Blvd. to the Rose Garden for the fourth BREAK.

5. Continue to Conservatory Drive and turn left. Cut through the park diagonally to reach the intersection of Stanton and Fulton. Turn north on Stanton and follow it to Geary. Cross over to Commonwealth and follow it north to California Pacific Medical Center for fifth BREAK.

6. Go east up California to Spruce St. and follow it north over a little hill. Drop down to Pacific St. and turn east up the Pacific St. hill. Continue to Pierce St. Turn north one block to Vallejo, then follow Vallejo east to Franklin. Follow Franklin north to Bay, Bay to Van Ness and north again to Aquatic Park.

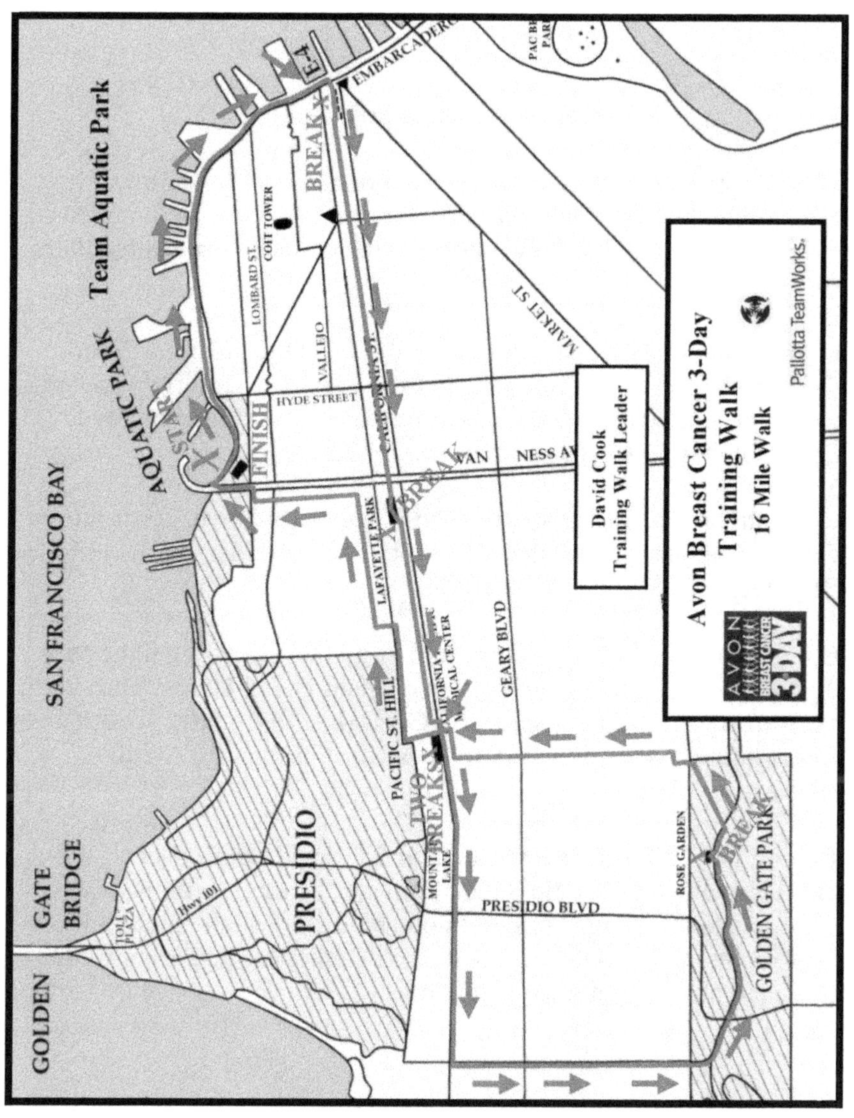
GOLDEN GATE BRIDGE
SAN FRANCISCO BAY
AQUATIC PARK
Team Aquatic Park
START
FINISH
BREAK
E-4
EMBARCADERO
COIT TOWER
LOMBARD ST.
VALLEJO
HYDE STREET
VAN NESS AV
MARKET ST
LAFAYETTE PARK
PACIFIC ST. HILL
GEARY BLVD
TWO BREAKS
PRESIDIO
Hwy 101
TOLL PLAZA
PRESIDIO BLVD
ROSE GARDEN
GOLDEN GATE PARK
David Cook
Training Walk Leader
Avon Breast Cancer 3-Day
Training Walk
16 Mile Walk
AVON BREAST CANCER 3·DAY
Pallotta TeamWorks

17 Mile Walk

Meet at Aquatic Park

1. Walk west through Fort Mason and Marina, then cross north and walk along the beach nearly to Fort Point. Turn uphill on Long Ave. to Lincoln Blvd. and follow it north to the Golden Gate Bridge Plaza and BREAK.

2. Follow Lincoln Blvd. all the way until it exits the Presidio. Veer right to 25th Ave. and follow it south to Clement. Turn right and go west on Clement to 40th Ave. Turn south a block to Geary Blvd. Follow it west to Cliff House for second BREAK.

3. Go south on Great Highway to John F. Kennedy Drive. Cross into Golden Gate Park and follow JFK to the Rose Garden for the third BREAK.

4. Continue to Conservatory Drive and turn left. Cut through the park diagonally to reach the intersection of Stanton and Fulton. Turn north on Stanton and follow it to Geary. Cross over to Commonwealth and follow it north to California Pacific Medical Center for fourth BREAK.

5. Go east up California to Spruce St. and follow it north over a little hill. Drop down to Pacific St. and turn east up the Pacific St. hill. Continue to Pierce St. Turn north one block to Vallejo, then follow Vallejo east to Franklin. Follow Franklin north to Bay, Bay to Van Ness and north again to Aquatic Park.

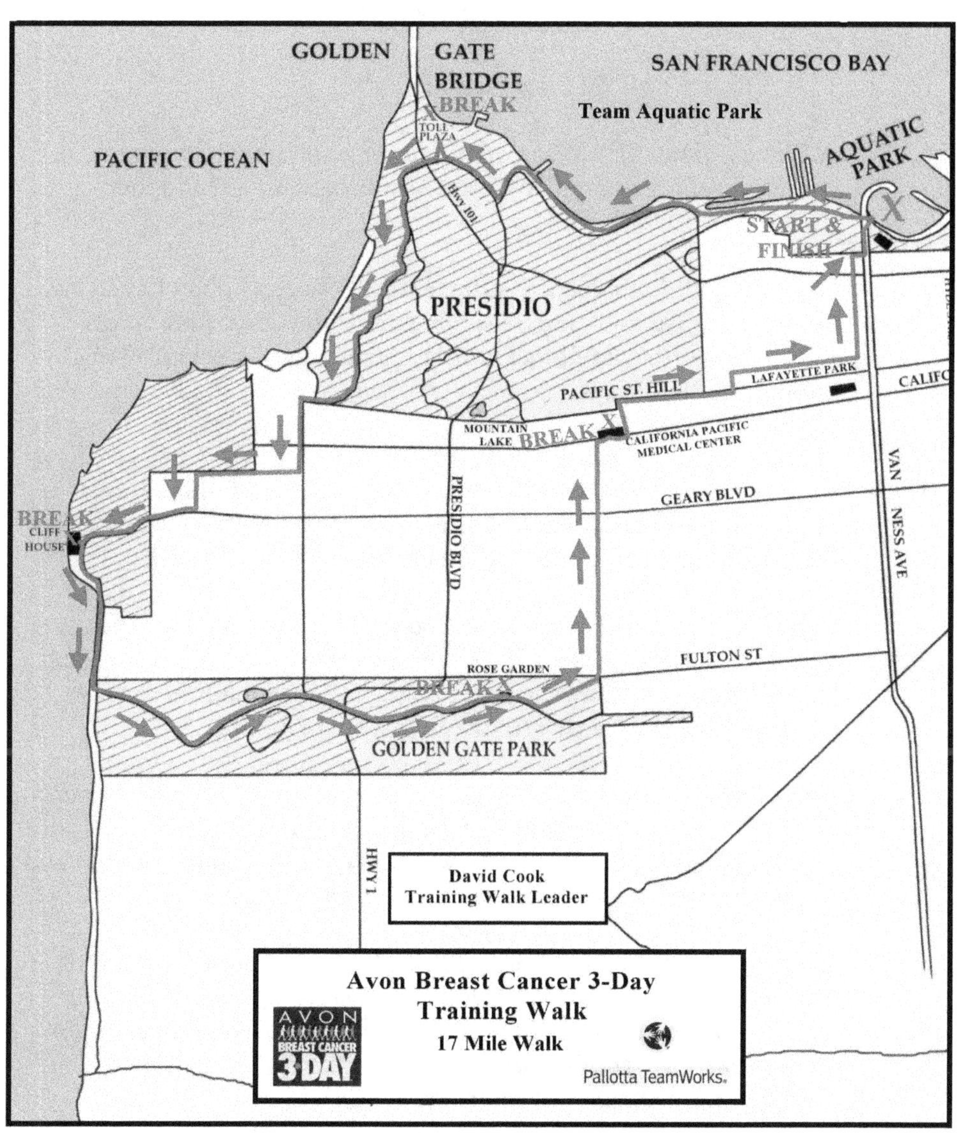
GOLDEN GATE BRIDGE
SAN FRANCISCO BAY
BREAK
TOLL PLAZA
Team Aquatic Park
PACIFIC OCEAN
AQUATIC PARK
Hwy 101
START & FINISH
PRESIDIO
LAFAYETTE PARK
PACIFIC ST. HILL
MOUNTAIN LAKE
BREAK
CALIFORNIA PACIFIC MEDICAL CENTER
VAN NESS AVE
PRESIDIO BLVD
GEARY BLVD
BREAK
CLIFF HOUSE
FULTON ST
ROSE GARDEN
BREAK
GOLDEN GATE PARK
HWY 1
David Cook
Training Walk Leader
Avon Breast Cancer 3-Day
Training Walk
17 Mile Walk
AVON
BREAST CANCER
3-DAY
Pallotta TeamWorks.

18 Mile Walk

Meet at Aquatic Park

1. Walk east along the Embarcadero, turning south with the street, just past Pier 39. Cross Embarcadero to Embarcadero 4, 2nd Floor (Lobby Level) for BREAK.

2. Walk through Embarcadero Center west between Lobby Level and Promenade (3rd Floor) to Sansome where you descend to Street Level. Jag north a half block to Clay St. and head west up a long hill through Chinatown. Continue all the way to Lafayette Park for the second BREAK.

3. Come south out of Lafayette Park to Sacramento. Follow it west to Spruce St., then jag south to California and follow it up the block to the California Pacific Medical Center for the third BREAK.

4. Continue west on California to 32nd Ave. Turn south one block to Clement and turn west again. Continue to 38th Ave. and turn south. Continue into Golden Gate Park, going east on John F. Kennedy Blvd. to the Rose Garden for the fourth BREAK.

5. Continue to Conservatory Drive and turn left. Cut through the park diagonally to reach the intersection of Stanton and Fulton. Turn north on Stanton and follow it to Geary. Cross over to Commonwealth and follow it north to California Pacific Medical Center for fifth BREAK.

6. Go east up California to Spruce St. and follow it north over a little hill. Drop down to Pacific St. and turn east up the Pacific St. hill. Continue to Pierce St. Turn north one block to Vallejo, then follow Vallejo east to Franklin. Follow Franklin north to Bay, Bay to Van Ness and north again to Aquatic Park.

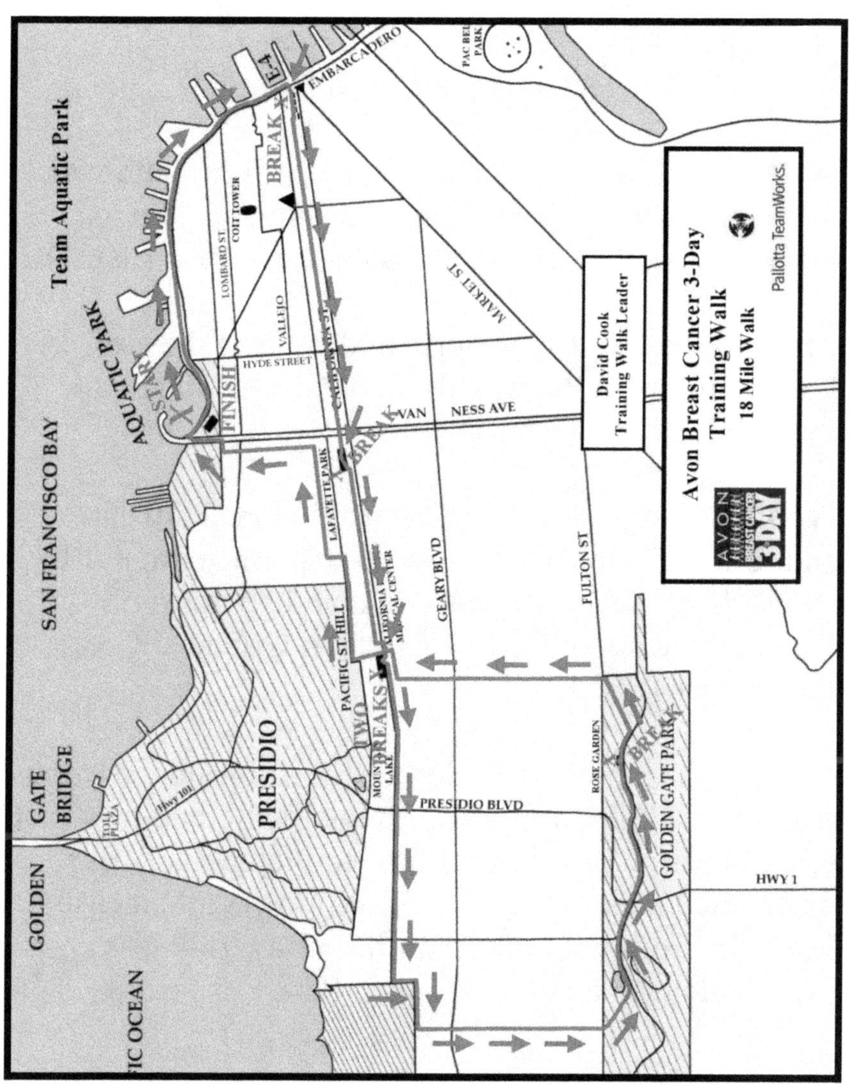
Team Aquatic Park
SAN FRANCISCO BAY
GOLDEN GATE BRIDGE
AQUATIC PARK
START
FINISH
HYDE STREET
VAN NESS AVE
BREAK
EMBARCADERO
E-4
COIT TOWER
LOMBARD ST
VALLEJO
MARKET ST
LAFAYETTE PARK
PACIFIC ST. HILL
GEARY BLVD
FULTON ST
PRESIDIO
TWO BREAKS
PRESIDIO BLVD
Hwy 101
TOLL PLAZA
ROSE GARDEN
GOLDEN GATE PARK
HWY 1
David Cook
Training Walk Leader
Avon Breast Cancer 3-Day
Training Walk
18 Mile Walk
Pallotta TeamWorks.
AVON BREAST CANCER 3-DAY

Bay to Breakers - Appx. 19 Miles

Meet at Aquatic Park

1. Walk east along the Embarcadero, turning south with the street, just past Pier 39. Cross Embarcadero to Embarcadero 4, 2nd Floor (Lobby Level) for BREAK.

2. Cross Market St. to the north and get into the crowd. Follow along all the way through Golden Gate Park to the ocean. BREAK.

3. Walk north on Great Highway to Fulton. Turn east and follow Fulton all the way to Stanton. Turn north and walk to Geary. Jag east a bit and go north on Commonwealth to California Pacific Medical Center for another BREAK.

4. Go east up California to Spruce St. and follow it north over a little hill. Drop down to Pacific St. and turn east up the Pacific St. hill. Continue to Pierce St. Turn north one block to Vallejo, then follow Vallejo east to Franklin. Follow Franklin north to Bay, Bay to Van Ness and north again to Aquatic Park.

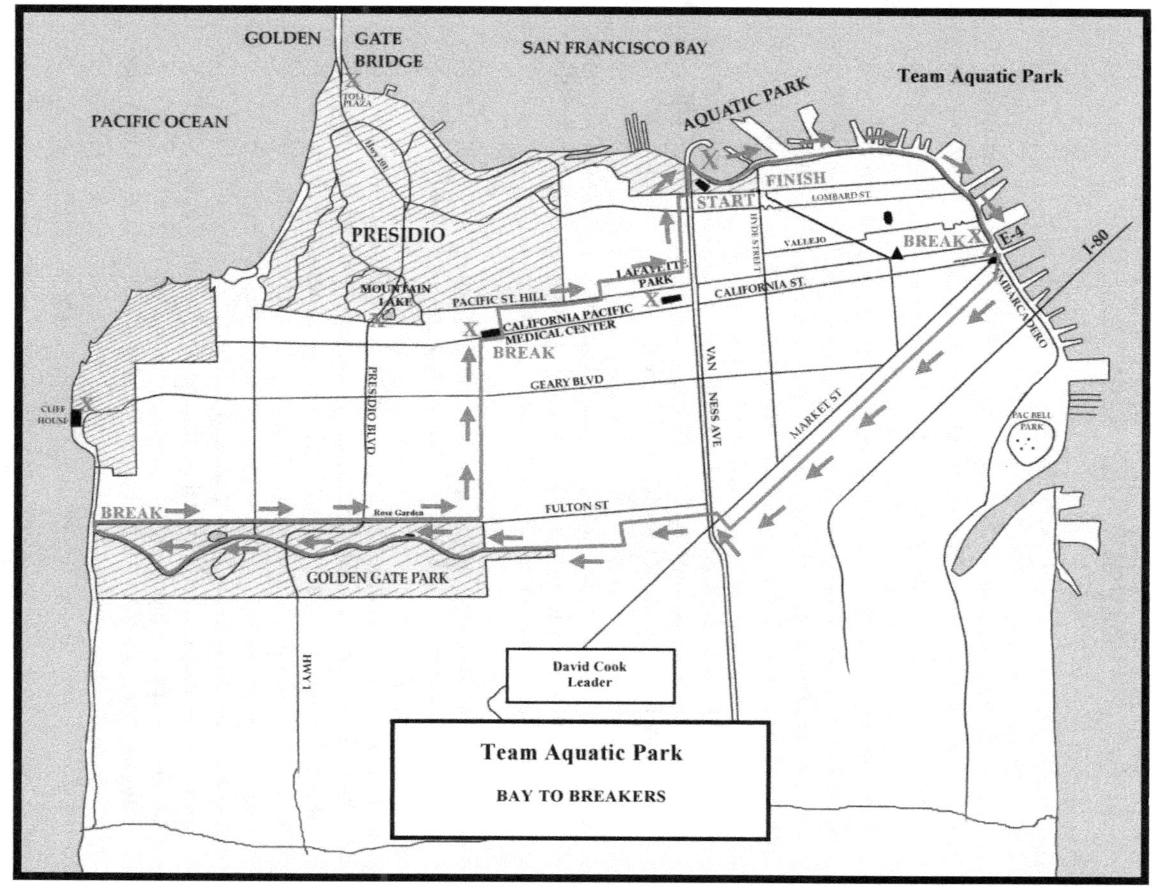
GOLDEN
GATE
BRIDGE
SAN FRANCISCO BAY
Team Aquatic Park
PACIFIC OCEAN
TOLL PLAZA
AQUATIC PARK
FINISH
START
LOMBARD ST.
PRESIDIO
HYDE STREET
VALLEJO
BREAK
E-4
I-80
LAFAYETTE PARK
MOUNTAIN LAKE
PACIFIC ST. HILL
CALIFORNIA ST.
CALIFORNIA PACIFIC MEDICAL CENTER
BREAK
EMBARCADERO
GEARY BLVD
PRESIDIO BLVD
VAN NESS AVE
MARKET ST
CLIFF HOUSE
PAC BELL PARK
BREAK
Rose Garden
FULTON ST
GOLDEN GATE PARK
HWY 1
David Cook
Leader
Team Aquatic Park
BAY TO BREAKERS

20 Mile Walk - Day 3 Sim

Meet at Aquatic Park

1. Walk east along the Embarcadero, turning south with the street, just past Pier 39. Cross Embarcadero to Embarcadero 4, 2nd Floor (Lobby Level) for BREAK.

2. Walk through Embarcadero Center west between Lobby Level and Promenade (3rd Floor) to Sansome where you descend to Street Level. Jag north a half block to Clay St. and head west up a long hill through Chinatown. Continue all the way to Lafayette Park for the second BREAK.

3. Come south out of Lafayette Park to Sacramento. Follow it west to Spruce St., then jag south to California and follow it up the block to the California Pacific Medical Center for the third BREAK.

4. Continue west on California to 32nd Ave. Turn south one block to Clement and turn west againto 40th Ave. Turn south a block to Geary Blvd. Follow it west to Cliff House for fourth BREAK

5 Go south on Great Highway to John F. Kennedy Drive. Cross into Golden Gate Park and follow JFK to the Rose Garden for the fifth BREAK.

6. Continue to Conservatory Drive and turn left. Cut through the park diagonally to reach the intersection of Stanton and Fulton. Turn north on Stanton and follow it to Geary. Cross over to Commonwealth and follow it north to California Pacific Medical Center for sixth BREAK.

7. Go east up California to Spruce St. and follow it north over a little hill. Drop down to Pacific St. and turn east up the Pacific St. hill. Continue to Pierce St. Turn north one block to Vallejo, then follow Vallejo east to Franklin. Follow Franklin north to Bay, Bay to Van Ness and north again to Aquatic Park.

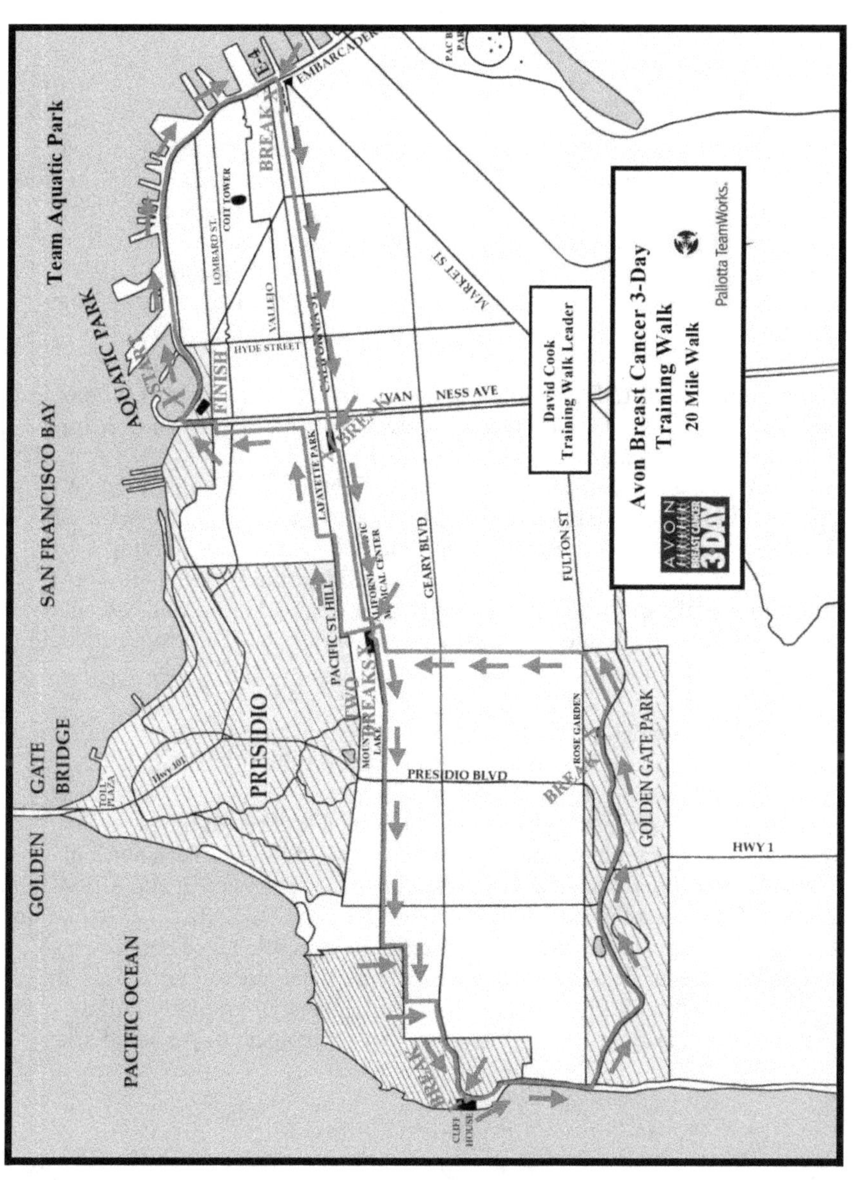
Avon Breast Cancer 3-Day
Training Walk
20 Mile Walk
David Cook
Training Walk Leader
Pallotta TeamWorks.
Team Aquatic Park
SAN FRANCISCO BAY
AQUATIC PARK
START
FINISH
GOLDEN GATE BRIDGE
TOLL PLAZA
Hwy 101
PACIFIC OCEAN
PRESIDIO
PACIFIC ST. HILL
LAFAYETTE PARK
LOMBARD ST.
COIT TOWER
VALLEJO
HYDE STREET
VAN NESS AVE
MARKET ST
GEARY BLVD
FULTON ST
PRESIDIO BLVD
ROSE GARDEN
GOLDEN GATE PARK
HWY 1
CLIFF HOUSE
E-4
BREAK

22 Mile Walk

Meet at Aquatic Park

1. Walk east along the Embarcadero, turning south with the street, just past Pier 39. Cross Embarcadero to Embarcadero 4, 2nd Floor (Lobby Level) for BREAK.... **2**. Walk through Embarcadero Center west between Lobby Level and Promenade (3rd Floor) to Sansome where you descend to Street Level. Jag north a half block to Clay St. and head west up a long hill through Chinatown. Continue all the way to Lafayette Park for the second BREAK.

3. Come south out of Lafayette Park to Sacramento. Follow it west to Spruce St., then jag south to California and follow it up the block to the California Pacific Medical Center for the third BREAK... **4**. Continue west to Arguello and turn north until you enter the Presidio. Continuing north past the golf course, follow the path left roughly following Arguello. You come out on Washington. Follow it to Battery Caulfield. Go south on BC until it becomes Wedemeyer. Follow that past the old Marine Hospital out of the Presidio to California St. Turn west on California to 32nd Ave. Turn south one block to Clement and turn west again to 40th Ave. Turn south a block to Geary Blvd. Follow it west to Cliff House for fourth BREAK

5 Go south on Great Highway to John F. Kennedy Drive. Cross into Golden Gate Park and follow JFK to the Rose Garden for the fifth BREAK.

6. Continue to Conservatory Drive and turn left. Cut through the park diagonally to reach the intersection of Stanton and Fulton. Turn north on Stanton and follow it to Geary. Cross over to Commonwealth and follow it north to California Pacific Medical Center for sixth BREAK... **7**. Go east up California to Spruce St. and follow it north over a little hill. Drop down to Pacific St. and turn east up the Pacific St. hill. Continue to Pierce St. Turn north one block to Vallejo, then follow Vallejo east to Franklin. Follow Franklin north to Bay, Bay to Van Ness and north again to Aquatic Park.

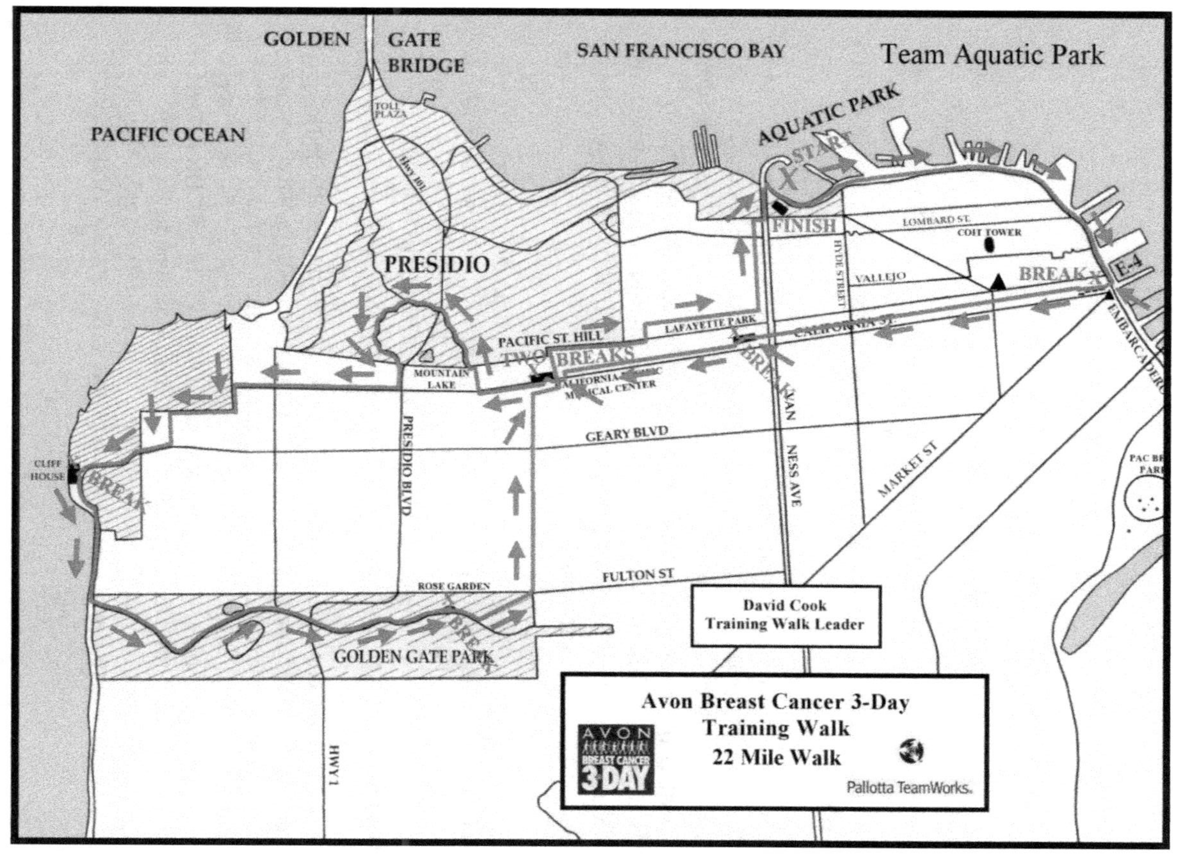
Team Aquatic Park
GOLDEN GATE BRIDGE
SAN FRANCISCO BAY
PACIFIC OCEAN
TOLL PLAZA
Hwy 101
AQUATIC PARK
START
FINISH
PRESIDIO
LOMBARD ST.
COIT TOWER
HYDE STREET
VALLEJO
BREAK
E-4
EMBARCADERO
LAFAYETTE PARK
CALIFORNIA ST.
PACIFIC ST. HILL
TWO BREAKS
MOUNTAIN LAKE
CALIFORNIA PACIFIC MEDICAL CENTER
BREAK
VAN NESS AVE
GEARY BLVD
MARKET ST
CLIFF HOUSE
BREAK
PRESIDIO BLVD
FULTON ST
ROSE GARDEN
BREAK
GOLDEN GATE PARK
David Cook
Training Walk Leader
Avon Breast Cancer 3-Day
Training Walk
22 Mile Walk
AVON BREAST CANCER 3DAY
Pallotta TeamWorks.
HWY 1

23 Mile Walk - Day 1 Sim

Meet at Aquatic Park

1. Walk east along the Embarcadero, turning south with the street, just past Pier 39. Cross Embarcadero to Embarcadero 4, 2nd Floor (Lobby Level) for BREAK.... **2**. Walk through Embarcadero Center west between Lobby Level and Promenade (3rd Floor) to Sansome where you descend to Street Level. Jag north a half block to Clay St. and head west up a long hill through Chinatown. Continue all the way to Lafayette Park for the second BREAK.

3. Come south out of Lafayette Park to Sacramento. Follow it west to Spruce St., then jag south to California and follow it up the block to the California Pacific Medical Center for the third BREAK... **4**. Go west on California to enter the Presidio on 14th Ave. Follow Wedemeyer north to Battery Caulfield to Washington and loop around the Presidio Golf Course to Arguello. Turn southwest behind driving range to Mountain Lake for fourth BREAK.

5. Continue west to Lake St. and follow it west to 25th Ave. Turn south two blocks to Clement and turn west again to 40th Ave. Turn south a block to Geary Blvd. Follow it west to Cliff House for fourth BREAK... **6**. Go south on Great Highway to John F. Kennedy Drive. Cross into Golden Gate Park and follow JFK to the Rose Garden for the fifth BREAK.

7. Continue to Conservatory Drive and turn left. Cut through the park diagonally to reach the intersection of Stanton and Fulton. Turn north on Stanton and follow it to Geary. Cross over to Commonwealth and follow it north to California Pacific Medical Center for sixth BREAK... **8**. Go east up California to Spruce St. and follow it north over a little hill. Drop down to Pacific St. and turn east up the Pacific St. hill. Continue to Pierce St. Turn north one block to Vallejo, then follow Vallejo east to Franklin. Follow Franklin north to Bay, Bay to Van Ness and north again to Aquatic Park.

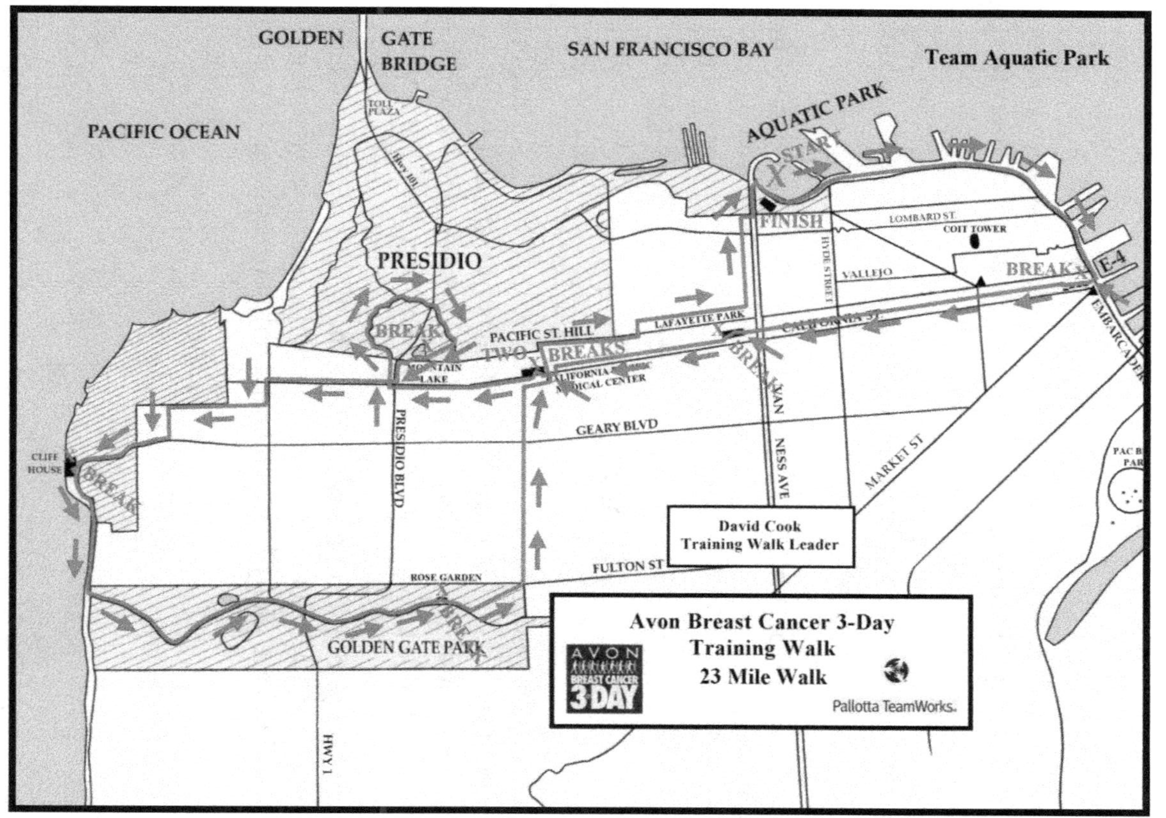
GOLDEN GATE BRIDGE
SAN FRANCISCO BAY
Team Aquatic Park
PACIFIC OCEAN
AQUATIC PARK
START
FINISH
TOLL PLAZA
Hwy 101
PRESIDIO
BREAK
PACIFIC ST. HILL
TWO BREAKS
LAFAYETTE PARK
CALIFORNIA ST.
LOMBARD ST.
COIT TOWER
VALLEJO
HYDE STREET
E-4
EMBARCADERO
MOUNTAIN LAKE
MEDICAL CENTER
VAN NESS AVE
PRESIDIO BLVD
GEARY BLVD
MARKET ST
CLIFF HOUSE
FULTON ST
ROSE GARDEN
GOLDEN GATE PARK
HWY 1
David Cook
Training Walk Leader
Avon Breast Cancer 3-Day
Training Walk
23 Mile Walk
AVON
BREAST CANCER
3-DAY
Pallotta TeamWorks.

Acknowledgements

Special thanks to Kat Cloran and the Gratitude Café and Bakery, Harlan Heald, Phyllis Moore, and Larry Reznicek for your food, insight, opinions, and (very grateful indeed) your sharp eyes!

Kevan Curren, thank you so much for your patience. I know it took years, but I finally finished it!

Lastly, love and deepest thanks to my sister, Patricia Kozak, for sticking with me through so many revisions.

Biography

Paul Wake Baker is a graduate of the University of Nebraska-Lincoln and a veteran of the United States Army. He has lived in many places but San Francisco and Santa Fe have been his favorites. He has written most of his life. It is a painful, difficult experience for him, but he has been stuck in it for quite some time now. He has written songs and performed publicly for most of his life, but is now a bit reclusive as he attempts to tidy up a few loose ends. If you feel expansive, wish him luck, because there are many loose ends and only one of him.

www.ingramcontent.com/pod-product-compliance
Lightning Source LLC
LaVergne TN
LVHW010559100826
845148LV00014B/2769